# Surgery for Chest Wall Deformities

Gary W. Raff • Shinjiro Hirose
Editors

# Surgery for Chest Wall Deformities

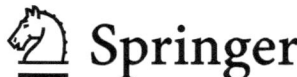 Springer

*Editors*
Gary W. Raff
Department of Surgery
University of California Davis
Sacramento, California, USA

Shinjiro Hirose
Division of Pediatric General,
   Thoracic, and Fetal Surgery
UC Davis Medical Center
Shriners Hospitals for
   Children—Northern California
Sacramento, California, USA

ISBN 978-3-319-43924-2      ISBN 978-3-319-43926-6   (eBook)
DOI 10.1007/978-3-319-43926-6

Library of Congress Control Number: 2016957344

Printed on acid-free paper

This Springer imprint is published by Springer Nature
The registered company is Springer International Publishing AG
The registered company address is: Gewerbestrasse 11, 6330 Cham, Switzerland

# Contents

1   **Surgical Anatomy of the Chest Wall** ........................ 1
Amy Rahm

2   **Pectus Excavatum** ..................................... 7
Yuen Julia Chen and Shinjiro Hirose

3   **Magnetic Mini-Mover Procedure for Pectus Excavatum** ....... 19
Claire Graves and Shinjiro Hirose

4   **Pectus Carinatum** ..................................... 27
Yuen Julia Chen and Shinjiro Hirose

5   **Anesthetic Considerations for Chest Wall Surgery** ........... 33
Rajvinder S. Dhamrait and Sundeep S. Tumber

6   **Poland's Syndrome** .................................... 47
Alessandro G. Cusano and Michael S. Wong

7   **Sternal Clefts and Anomalies** ........................... 71
Luis Godoy and Gary Raff

8   **Chest Wall Tumors** .................................... 83
Sabrina A. Oldfield and Elizabeth A. David

9   **Role of Nurse Practitioners in Chest Wall Clinics
as a Model for Care** .................................... 101
Mary Zanobini, Barbara Goebel, Amy B. Powne,
Robyn H. Lao, and Karen S. Brand

**Index** ...................................................... 107

# Contributors

**Karen S. Brand, R.N., M.S.N., C.P.N.P.-AC.** Shriners Hospital of Northern California, Sacramento, CA, USA

**Yuen Julia Chen, M.D.** Department of Surgery, Mount Sinai Medical Center, New York, NY, USA

**Alessandro G. Cusano, M.D.** Department of surgery, Division of Plastic Surgery, University of California Davis Medical Center, Sacramento, CA, USA

**Elizabeth A. David, M.D. F.A.C.S.** Section of General Thoracic Surgery, Department of Surgery, UC Davis Medical Center, Sacramento, CA, USA
Heart Lung Vascular Center, David Grant Medical Center, Sacramento, CA, USA

**Rajvinder S. Dhamrait, BM, DCH, FCARCSI, FRCA** Department of Anesthesiology and Pain Medicine, University of California, Davis School of Medicine, UC Davis Children's Hospital, Sacramento, CA, USA

**Luis Godoy, M.D.** Department of Surgery, University of California, Davis Medical Center, Sacramento, CA, USA

**Barbara Goebel, N.P., R.N.F.A.** Pediatric Heart Center, University of California, Davis Children's Hospital, Sacramento, CA, USA

**Claire Graves** Department of Surgery, Columbia University, New York, NY, USA

**Shinjiro Hirose, M.D.** Division of Pediatric General, Thoracic, and Fetal Surgery, UC Davis Medical Center, Shriners Hospitals for Children—Northern California, Sacramento, CA, USA

**Robyn H. Lao, R.N., M,S.N., D.N.P., C.P.N.P.-AC** University of California, Davis Children's Hospital, Sacramento, CA, USA

**Sabrina A. Oldfield, M.D.** Section of General Thoracic Surgery, Department of Surgery, UC Davis Medical Center, Sacramento, CA, USA

**Amy B. Powne, R.N., C.N.S** University of California, Davis Children's Hospital, Sacramento, CA, USA

**Amy Rahm, M.D.** Division of Pediatric Cardiothoracic Surgery, University of California, Davis Medical Center, Sacramento, CA, USA

**Gary Raff, M.D.** Department of Surgery, Pediatric Heart Center, University of California, Davis, Sacramento, CA, USA

**Sundeep S. Tumber, D.O.** Shriners Hospitals for Children—Northern California, Sacramento, CA, USA

**Michael S. Wong, M.D.** Department of Surgery, University of California, Davis Medical Center, Sacramento, CA, USA

**Mary Zanobini, N.P., R.N.F.A.** Pediatric Heart Center, University of California, Davis Children's Hospital, Sacramento, CA, USA

Amy Rahm

## Sternum

The sternum is comprised of three components, the manubrium, sternal body, and xiphoid (Fig. 1.1). The superior most portion of the sternum is the manubrium which abuts the clavicles bilaterally through shallow facets. The suprasternal notch is the depression along the upper border of the manubrium between the two clavicular heads that is easily identifiable on physical exam. It denotes the level of the second thoracic vertebrae. The cartilaginous portion of the first ribs also articulate with the manubrium via bilateral costal incisura. The second costal cartilages articulate with the inferior–lateral surface of the manubrium as well as the superior–lateral surface of the sternal body via separate synovial joints. The final articulation site of the manubrium is the manubriosternal joint, also known as the sternal angle because of the steeper angulation of the sternal body in relation to the manubrium. Identifying this structure on the surface anatomy provides identification of the second intercostal space just lateral to its location as well as the level of bifurcation of the trachea, the upper border of

the atria of the heart, and the level of the fourth to fifth thoracic vertebrae. Both, the articular surface of the manubrium and the sternal body, are covered with hyaline cartilage allowing for flexible movement of the sternal body and connecting ribs during respiration. This joint may ossify in some conditions such as Pouter pigeon chest, resulting in decreased chest wall compliance and abnormal contour of the chest wall. The muscular attachments to the manubrium include the sternohyoid, sternothyroid, and sternocleidomastoid muscles as well as a portion of the pectoralis major muscle.

During development, the sternum consists of six sternebrae (Fig. 1.2). During late adolescence, the central four segments fuse to form the sternal body. The sternal body is bordered bilaterally by the articulation of the second through seventh costal cartilages. A common variant in females is the joining of the facets for the sixth and seventh costal cartilages. The lateral sternal border also attaches to the internal intercostal muscles and anterior intercostal membrane while the pectoralis major muscle attaches along the anterior–lateral surface.

The xiphoid process is a cartilaginous structure that attaches inferiorly to the sternal body along with connections to the costal margin of the seventh rib via the costoxiphoid ligament and a direct attachment to the rectus sheath. It is noted to be variable in length and structure with the most common variants being bifid or perfo-

A. Rahm, M.D. (✉)
Division of Pediatric Cardiothoracic Surgery,
University of California, Davis Medical Center,
2221 Stockton Blvd. Suite 2112, Sacramento,
CA 95817, USA
e-mail: amyrahm42812@gmail.com

© Springer International Publishing Switzerland 2017
G.W. Raff, S. Hirose (eds.), *Surgery for Chest Wall Deformities*,
DOI 10.1007/978-3-319-43926-6_1

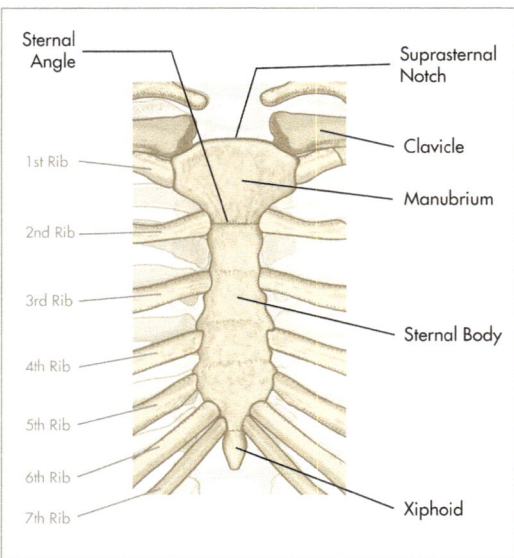

**Fig. 1.1** Anterior view of sternum with clavicular and costal cartilage attachments. Surface landmarks denoted (suprasternal notch and sternal angle)

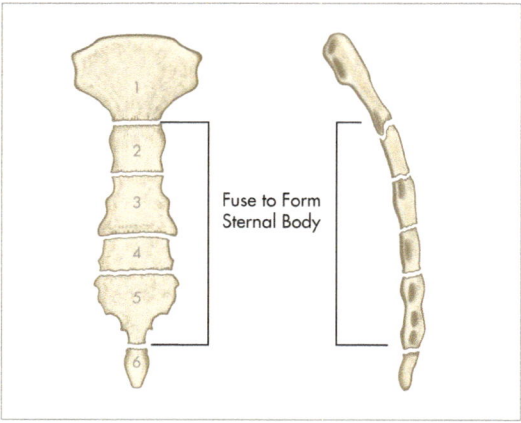

**Fig. 1.2** Developing sternum which consists of six separate sternabrae. The central four segments fuse during adolescence

rated. The xiphoid process is occasionally prominent enough to be seen on physical exam as a protrusion at the inferior border of the sternum.

## Ribs

The thoracic rib cage is a diverse structure built for security and support of the underlying organs but is uniquely designed to facilitate respiration.

There are 12 paired ribs along with their associated costal cartilages that develop from the costal process of each individual thoracic vertebrae. During development, rib pairs migrate superiorly so that they not only abut their original vertebra but also the one immediately cephalad. This migration affects ribs 2 through 9 and occasionally the tenth rib. The cephalic migration of the vertebral end relative to the sternal end of the ribs explains the characteristic shape of the rib cage.

Ribs 1 through 7, referred to as true ribs, articulate with the manubrium or sternum while ribs 8 through 10, known as false ribs, articulate with the costal cartilage of the adjacent ribs. Ribs 11 and 12 do not have an anterior articulation point and are therefore free floating (Fig. 1.3).

Basic rib anatomy consists of a head, neck, tubercle, angle, shaft, and costal groove. The head of a typical rib articulates at two points, the superior costal facet of the thoracic vertebra of the same number and the inferior costal facet of the thoracic vertebra just cephalad. An articular capsule surrounds the head of each rib and is further attached to the vertebra via the radiate ligament. The tubercule articulates with the transverse process of the adjacent vertebra along with the presence of multiple costotransverse ligaments for added support. As you follow the contour of the bony rib to the end of the shaft, you reach the costochondral joint where the bony rib and cartilage are securely attached via the intertwining of periosteum and perichondrium. The attachment of the first ribs is through synchondroses or cartilaginous joints and are therefore immobile while the second through seventh rib pairs articulate with the sternum via synovial joints that allow for movement during respiration. These joints are reinforced by sternocostal ligaments. The costal groove lies along the inferior surface and houses the intercostal neurovascular bundle (Fig. 1.4).

Ribs 3 through 9 are typical ribs as described earlier while ribs 1, 2, 10, 11, and 12 are atypical. The first rib is a short, flat rib that is much wider and more curved than those previously described. Its head has only one facet for articulation with the body of the first thoracic vertebrae and the prominent tubercle forms a synovial joint with the transverse process. Anteriorly, the first rib is

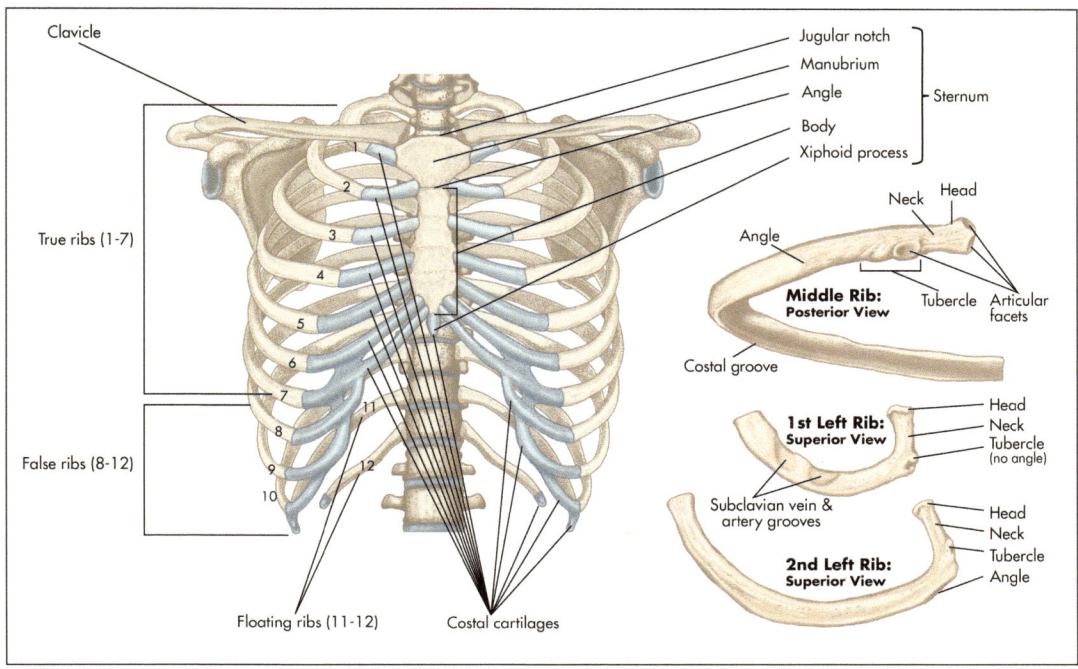

**Fig. 1.3**  Anterior view of the bony thorax and pectoral girdle.  True, false and floating ribs are denoted.  Insert contains images of a typical rib and the first rib

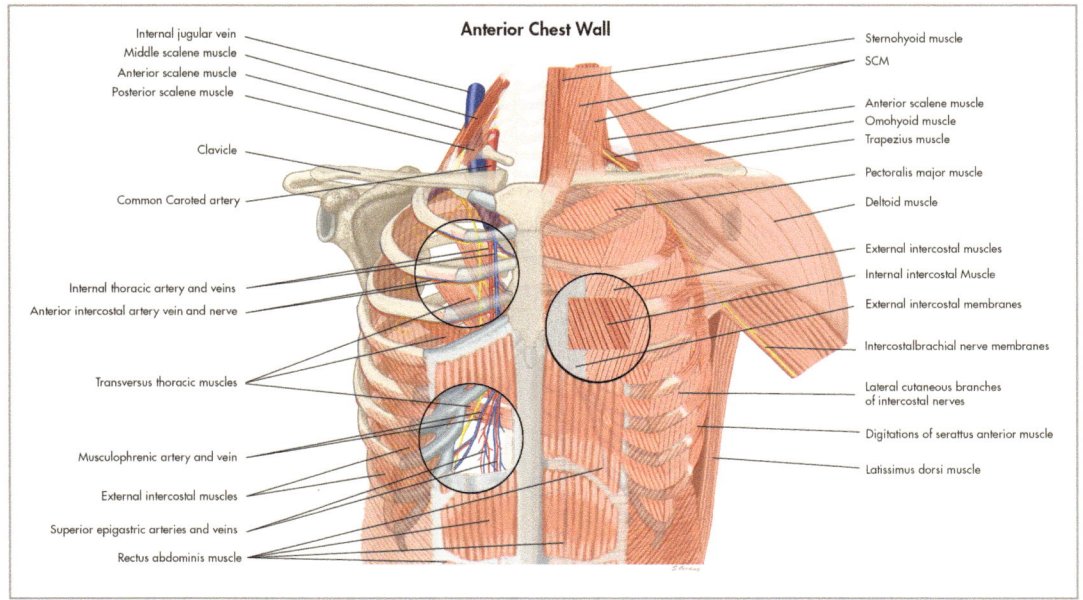

**Fig. 1.4**  Anterior chest wall showing muscular attachments and neurovascular structures

secured to the manubrium via a synchondrosis and the clavicle by the costoclavicular ligament. It has attachments from the anterior, middle, and posterior scalene muscles as well as the serratus anterior, subclavius, and erector spinae muscles. The subclavian artery and vein cross over the first ribs near the middle of the shaft and under the clavicles bilaterally. The second rib is unique in that it has a large tuberosity for attachment of the serratus anterior muscle and a poorly developed costal groove. The head of ribs 10–12 articulates with the corresponding thoracic vertebrae via one facet. Ribs 11 and 12 are further distinguished by lacking a neck, angle, and costal groove. They also do not articulate with the corresponding transverse process.

There are several types of rib variants of little conscience such as the bifid or forked rib, fusion of two or more ribs, and bridge formation between two ribs. These conditions occur in less than 1 % of the population and may have a female as well as a right-sided predilection. They are typically asymptomatic but may be associated with musculoskeletal pain or intercostal nerve entrapment. Bifid ribs are also associated with Gorlin syndrome (nevoid basal cell carcinoma). Up to 16 % of the population may exhibit a short rib described as a foreshortened midthoracic rib arch. It is asymptomatic and more commonly identified on the right side. A cervical rib, which arises from the seventh cervical vertebra is present in approximately 0.5 % of the population and is more common in females. Although it is typically asymptomatic, a cervical rib is the most important anatomic rib variant because it can produce thoracic outlet syndrome.

## Intercostal Muscles and the Intercostal Space

There are a multitude of surgical procedures that are performed on the chest wall and within the mediastinum and thorax which require precise knowledge of the musculoskeletal and neurovascular anatomy. Entry into the thorax for either tube thoracostomy or a surgical intervention requires the intercostal space to be traversed. Understanding the interspaces between the ribs are wider anteriorly due to the previously described upward transition of the vertebrae during development, is helpful when planning a surgical intervention. The ribs are connected by intercostal muscles and membranes (Figure 1.4). The outermost layer consists of the external intercostal muscles that arise from the sharp undersurface of the superior rib. The external intercostal muscles course inferomedially and insert on the smooth upper surface of the inferior rib. Where the bony rib transitions to costal cartilage, the external intercostal muscle is replaced by the external intercostal membrane. The next layer is composed of the internal intercostal muscles. These muscles originate from the lip of the costal groove of ribs 1–11 and insert on the smooth upper surface of the next rib. They course in an inferolateral trajectory and extend from the sternum to the angle of each rib. From the angle of the rib to the spine, the muscle is replaced with the internal intercostal membrane.

Paired internal thoracic arteries are found running longitudinally approximately 1 cm lateral to the sternum, along with two veins (venae comitantes). This vascular bundle sits just posterior to the internal intercostal muscles and anterior to the transversus thoracic muscles (anterior division of the innermost muscles) that extends from the underside of the sternum to the costal cartilages of ribs 2–6. The internal thoracic artery arises from the subclavian artery and branches into the superior epigastric and musculophrenic arteries after giving rise to each anterior intercostal artery that resides within the costal grooves. The posterior intercostal arteries arise from the thoracic aorta except within the first and second interspaces. At this location they are branches off the supreme intercostal artery from the costocervical trunk of the subclavian artery. The intercostal artery is accompanied by a vein and nerve within the costal groove. They are oriented superior to inferior, vein–artery–nerve (VAN). This neurovascular bundle sits between the internal intercostal muscles and the anterolateral portion of the innermost intercostal muscles. As the neurovascular bundle travels more posteriorly, it sits within the endothoracic fascia just deep to the internal intercostal membrane which allows it to be visible from within the chest during surgical procedures.

The intercostal nerves provide motor control of various muscles, such as the external/internal intercostal muscles, innermost intercostal muscles, and the serratus posterior inferior/superior muscles as well as sensory perception along the parietal pleura and skin. The first and second intercostal nerves innervate the upper limb as well as the thoracic wall. Intercostal nerves 6–11 not only innervate the thoracic wall but also the abdominal wall. Due to the overlapping innervation along the thoracic wall, it is uncommon to have postoperative paresthesia unless multiple intercostal nerves are injured. Because the intercostal nerves rest within the costal groove along the inferior border of the ribs, it is possible to enter the thoracic cavity along the superior margin of a rib and therefore avoid injury to the neurovascular bundle.

handle fashion. Accessory muscles are activated during forced inspiration and include the serratus anterior, pectoralis major and minor, trapezius, levator scapulae, rhomboids, and serratus posterior superior muscles. By increasing the dimensions of the chest wall during inspiration, a negative intra-thoracic pressure is created to draw air into the lungs. Relaxation of the diaphragm, elastic recoil of the lung, and contraction of the internal intercostal muscles lead to passive expiration. Accessory muscles of expiration include the rectus abdominis, external obliques, internal obliques, transversus thoracic, serratus posterior inferior, quadratus lumborum. Function of the upper extremities is controlled by the various muscles attached to the clavicle, scapula, and humerus. It is possible for some of these muscles to be absent such as in Poland's syndrome where the pectoralis major muscle is missing on one side of the body along with ipsilateral hand abnormalities.

## Muscles and Physiology of the Chest Wall

The muscles attached to the chest involved in respiratory function are divided into two categories, inspiratory and expiratory. The primary muscles of inspiration during relaxed breathing are the diaphragm and external intercostals. The diaphragm is attached to the xiphoid process, lower six ribs bilaterally and the lumbar vertebrae giving rise to the central tendon. During quiet inspiration the central tendon moves very little but during forced inspiration it is displaced downward up to four inches. The external intercostals function in respiration by elevating the ribs in a bucket handle fashion. The sternocleidomastoids and scalene muscles raise the sternum and upper ribs in a pump

## Suggested Readings

Blevins CE. Anatomy of the thorax. In: Shields TW et al., editors. General thoracic surgery, vol. 1. 6th ed. Philadelphia: Lippincott Williams & Wilkins; 2005. p. 3–15.

Clemens MW, Evans KK, et al. Introduction to chest wall reconstruction: anatomy and physiology of the chest and indications for chest wall reconstruction. Semin Plast Surg. 2011;25(1):5–15.

Kurihara Y, Yakushiji YK, et al. The ribs: anatomic and radiologic considerations. Radiographics. 1999;19(1): 105–19.

Naidu B, Rajesh PB. Relevant surgical anatomy of the chest wall. Thorac Surg Clin. 2010;20(4):453–63.

Shahani R. Anatomy of the thorax. In: Sellke FW et al., editors. Sabiston & spencer: surgery of the chest, vol. 1. 7th ed. Philadelphia: Elsevier Saunders; 2005. p. 3–18.

## Yuen Julia Chen and Shinjiro Hirose

## Introduction

Pectus excavatum, "funnel chest," is characterized by a depression of the sternum and the lower costal cartilages resulting in a decreased anteroposterior diameter of the chest. Pectus excavatum accounts for more than 90 % of all congenital chest wall deformities [1] and is a relatively common deformity, occurring between 0.1 and 0.8 per 100 persons [2]. There is a male predominance of 5:1 [3] and it is more common in Caucasians than Hispanic and African American populations [1].

## Historical

The first documented case of pectus excavatum occurred in the sixteenth century by French naturalist-botanist Johann Bauhinusa who

Y.J. Chen, M.D.
Department of Surgery, Mount Sinai Medical Center, New York, NY, USA
e-mail: juchen@ucdavis.edu

S. Hirose, M.D. (✉)
Division of Pediatric General, Thoracic, and Fetal Surgery, UC Davis Medical Center, Shriners Hospitals for Children—Northern California, Sacramento, CA, USA
e-mail: shirose@ucdavis.edu

described a case of "a severe form of funnel chest in a patient with extensive pressure on the lung, shortness of breath, and paroxysmal coughing" [4, 5]. Recently, however, excavated graves from Hungary identified fossilized sternums demonstrating the characteristic deformity that date back to as early as the tenth century [6]. In the nineteenth century numerous case reports followed with the prescribed treatment being "fresh air, breathing exercises, aerobic activities, and lateral pressure" [7].

The first repair was reported in 1911 by Meyer in which the rib cartilage was removed and analyzed in a patient with pectus excavatum [8]. In 1913, Sauerbruch described successful patient outcomes with a more aggressive technique of excising an entire section of the anterior chest wall to correct the deformity. In the 1920s, Sauerbruch then performed the first pectus repair using bilateral costal cartilage resection and sternal osteotomy [9]. Twenty years later, this would be the basis of the technique popularized by Dr. Mark Ravitch. In 1949, he described performing an open subperichondrial resection of the lower costal cartilages and a wedge osteotomy of the sternum to treat pectus excavatum. This became known as the Ravitch repair and the gold standard for decades to follow [10]. The procedure was further modified in the 1950s to use a short support bar or strut to augment the repair [7]. While popular, the modified Ravitch repair is not without its flaws, and throughout the 1990s multiple reports of complications including cardiac perforation, acquired Jeune Syndrome (asphyxiating thoracic chondrodystrophy), migration of the support bar, and laceration of the phrenic artery were reported.

As early as 1954, Judet introduced the concept of sternal turnover as a treatment methodology for pectus excavatum. This technique was utilized in Japan by Wada et al. in 1970 [11]; however, it was never widely adopted due to the high morbidity associated with sternal infection and necrosis. The concept of focusing on modifying the sternal structure was revisited in 1997 by Dr. Donald Nuss who reported a minimally invasive approach to correct the defect without removal of the costal cartilages in his 10 year series of 42 patients with pectus excavatum [12]. Rather than using surgical resection to mold the sternum, Nuss described using an internal stainless steel brace to correct the anterior chest wall depression.

Today, both the Nuss and modified Ravitch procedure are used for the surgical treatment of pectus excavatum, and identifying novel surgical techniques remains an area of active device innovation with new approaches in current clinical trials.

## Embryology and Anatomy

The trunk is developed from embryonic mesoderm and consists of muscles, ribs, costal cartilages, and the sternum. The musculature of the chest wall derives from myotomes formed in the fourth week of development. The ribs are formed during the fifth week arising from the thoracic vertebrae and develop towards the ventral body wall where they fuse with the sternum in the sixth week. The sternum develops from two lateral mesenchymal bands that fuse in a cranial to caudal direction. Ossification of the sternum begins at 6 months of age and is typically completed at the 12th year [4, 7].

The skeletal structure of the anterior chest consists of the sternum, which is made of the manubrium, sternal body and xiphoid process, and the 12 sets of bony ribs that articulate at the manubrium, sternum, and costal cartilages. The manubrium is located at the level of T3 and T4 and is the widest and thickest of the three sternal bones. The manubrium and sternal body lie in slightly different planes so that their junction at the manubriosternal joint projects anteriorly. The body of the sternum is located at T5–T9 and the xiphoid is the smallest and thinnest bone. The first seven ribs are true ribs and attach to the sternum and manubrium directly. The ribs and sternum connect at a hyaline cartilage joint known as the costochondral joint. The first pair of ribs articulates through a cartilaginous joint and is relatively immobile while the second to seventh pairs of costal cartilages articulate with the sternum at synovial joints that are able to move during respiration. The eighth to tenth ribs are false ribs and attach anteriorly via the costal cartilage where the ribs and cartilage are connected through their overlying periosteum and perichondrium. The 11th and 12th ribs are floating ribs and remain unattached anteriorly [13] (Fig. 2.1).

## Pathophysiology

The etiology of pectus excavatum remains unknown. There is a strong familial tendency with up to 43 % of presenting cases with a positive family history [14–16]; however, the exact genetic link is yet to be elucidated, and the inheritance pattern is likely multifactorial [17–19]. Pectus excavatum can be a part of many genetic syndromes, the most frequently observed being Marfan Syndrome and Noonan Syndrome [20]; however, less than 1 % of patients with pectus excavatum have an underlying connective tissue disorder [21].

There have been many historical theories regarding the pathogenesis of pectus excavatum including abnormal in utero diaphragmatic development, abnormal embryonic positioning resulting in increased intrauterine pressure on the sternum, and the sequelae of systemic diseases such as syphilis and rickets [4]. Current hypotheses on the etiology of pectus excavatum focus on abnormal metabolism and overgrowth at the sternocostal cartilage resulting in weakness and

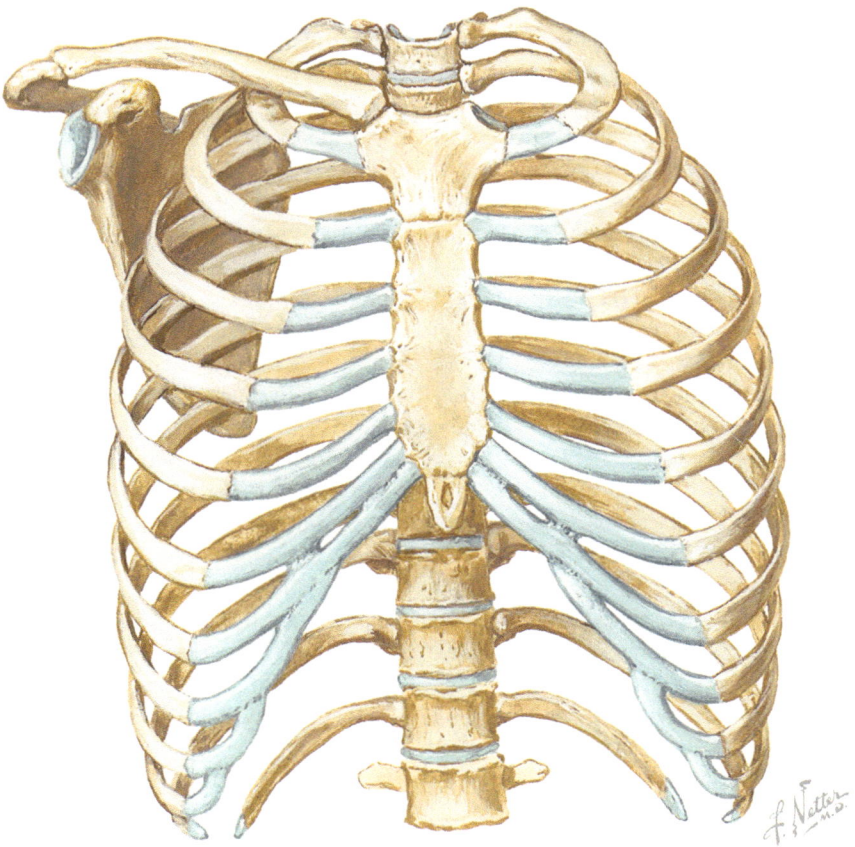

**Fig. 2.1** Chest wall anatomy (Netters)

instability at the joint [22]. Histological analysis of the sternocostal cartilage in patients with pectus excavatum reveals evidence of premature aging of the cartilage, abnormalities in the trace element content, namely decreased zinc, and decreased chondrocyte activity [23–25]. Relative to control specimen, cartilages from patients with pectus excavatum demonstrate decreased biomechanical stability, which is hypothesized to be the result of disordered arrangement and distribution of collagen [26].

## Presentation

Pectus excavatum can be present at birth; however, it is not typically recognized until early childhood and adolescence when patients experi-

ence rapid growth and the severity of the depression becomes more visible. For most patients there is little resulting effect on physiology but the physical appearance can lead to psychological distress and represents a significant indication for treatment.

## Clinical Features

Many patients who present with pectus excavatum are active and otherwise healthy appearing with only a visible anatomic defect as their chief complaint. Physical features include visible depression of the lower sternum with varying asymmetry of the chest wall. The deformity can be present in many different configurations with the most common being a cup-shaped concavity. The cup shape is usually well defined and deep, involving the lower end of the sternum. When the upper costal cartilages are involved, patients present with a broader and more extensive depression that is typically more severe. Patients with pectus excavatum often also have a classic posture associated with the anomaly. They are typically tall and thin with sloped ribs and rounded shoulders and a protuberant appearing abdomen. There is also a high association with scoliosis [27–29]. If symptomatic, the most common symptoms reported are nonspecific precordial chest pain, decreased exercise tolerance, frequent respiratory infections, asthma, and social anxiety regarding body image resulting in psychological distress [4].

## Cardiopulmonary Features

A systolic ejection murmur is frequently observed in patients with pectus excavatum and accentuated after exercise. This murmur is likely due to the decrease in proximity between the sternum and the pulmonary artery allowing transmission of a flow murmur. EKG abnormalities can be seen due to the abnormal configuration of the chest wall that displaces the heart towards the left [30].

As a structural abnormality of the chest wall, pectus excavatum can theoretically result in abnormal respiratory mechanics as well as cardiopulmonary impairment secondary to compression of the thoracic cavity. However, there are many authors who do not believe that pectus excavatum causes any cardiopulmonary impairment. Clinically, nonetheless, there is a general consensus that following surgical repair patients demonstrate increased exercise tolerance and stamina [30].

## Pulmonary Function Studies

Koumbourlis and Stolar [31] performed a comprehensive analysis of patterns of lung growth and function in 103 patients with idiopathic pectus excavatum. They found that there was a high prevalence of lower airway obstruction resulting in a pattern of obstructive lung disease rather than restrictive lung disease. They noted differences in lung function among different age groups; however, there was no evidence that the pectus deformity results in worsening lung growth or function as patients grow older.

A recent prospective multicenter study [32] of 327 pectus patients found a relatively small decrease in lung function studies preoperatively compared to normal with postsurgical improvement of approximately 6–10 %. Those with more severe anatomic depression had greater postoperative improvement in lung function. Preoperative and postoperative exercise pulmonary function tests showed that after surgery patients had a 10.2 % increase in maximum oxygen uptake and a 19 % increase in oxygen pulse. Although the differences between preoperative and postoperative pulmonary function tests were statistically significant, the authors still concluded that these changes were only modest in magnitude after repair.

Finally, a meta-analysis published in 2006 [33] of 12 studies with 313 pectus patients concluded that operative repair of pectus excavatum resulted in no statistically significant change in pulmonary function. Despite the multitude of studies published on this topic, there is still no consensus on the impact of the deformity on any objective measure of pulmonary physiology.

## Cardiovascular Studies

In patients with pectus excavatum, the posterior depression of the sternum can result in an anterior depression of the right ventricle and displacement of the heart to the left [30]. Studies with small sample sizes suggest that patients with this compression have decreased stroke volume and cardiac output compared to normal controls and are limited in their ability to increase stroke volume with exercise [34]. The incidence of mitral valve prolapse is higher in pectus patients (17–65 %) as compared to the normal pediatric population (1 %). This is theorized to be the result of cardiac compression as postoperative studies suggest that up to 50 % of mitral valve prolapse resolves after pectus repair [35, 36]. Dysarrythmias such as first degree heart block, right bundle branch block, and Wolff–Parkinson–White are also common with an incidence of 16% in the pectus excavatum population [7].

A meta-analysis published in 2006 [37] examined pre- and postoperative cardiovascular function in 169 pectus patients. The authors concluded based on the eight studies that met their eligibility criteria that on average, quantitative measures of cardiovascular function improved by greater than one half standard deviation following surgical repair. Controversy, however, remains, as a subsequent meta-analysis published in 2007 [38] reviewed the same literature and concluded that there was no reliable documentation of improvement in cardiac function after pectus repair.

## Initial Assessment

The evaluation of a patient with pectus excavatum, like any other chest wall deformity, begins with a thorough history and physical exam. A careful assessment of the severity of the defect, symptomatology, and potential for limitations on cardiac and pulmonary physiology should be considered. Specifically, attention should be paid towards exercise tolerance, pain along the sternal border and lower costal margins, and psychological distress from body image issues. On physical exam, the depth of the defect and evidence of rotation should be documented [21].

Imaging studies can further assist in anatomic assessment and documentation of chest wall dimensions. These tests are particularly valuable for preoperative planning. There have been studies advocating that a routine chest radiograph be the sole imaging required for preoperative assessment [39]; however, the majority of patients undergo computed tomography (CT) scan of the chest. magnetic resonance imaging (MRI) may be used in patients where radiation exposure is a significant concern; however, CT is typically considered a more favorable imaging modality given its improved visualization of bony detail compared to MRI [7].

There are a variety of scoring indices to assess the severity of sternal depression, but the most widely accepted is the Haller index. The Haller index is calculated radiographically by dividing the transverse breadth of the chest by the narrowest sternovertebral distance. A Haller index greater than 3.25 is considered to be indicative of a severe defect [40] (Fig. 2.2).

Almost all patients undergo pulmonary function testing prior to operative repair; however, normal results do not preclude operative intervention. Patients who have a history of palpitations should have a 24-h electrocardiogram looking for arrhythmias as well as an echocardiogram to evaluate for possible mitral valve prolapse.

## Indications for Operative Repair

Factors that determine operative candidacy include anatomic changes, physiologic limitations, and psychological distress. The indications

**Fig. 2.2** Haller index

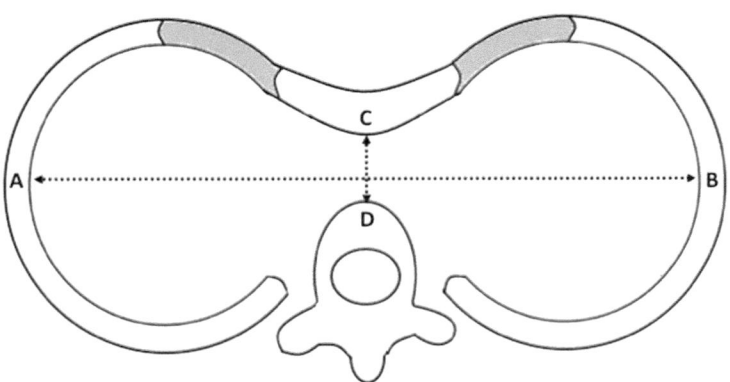

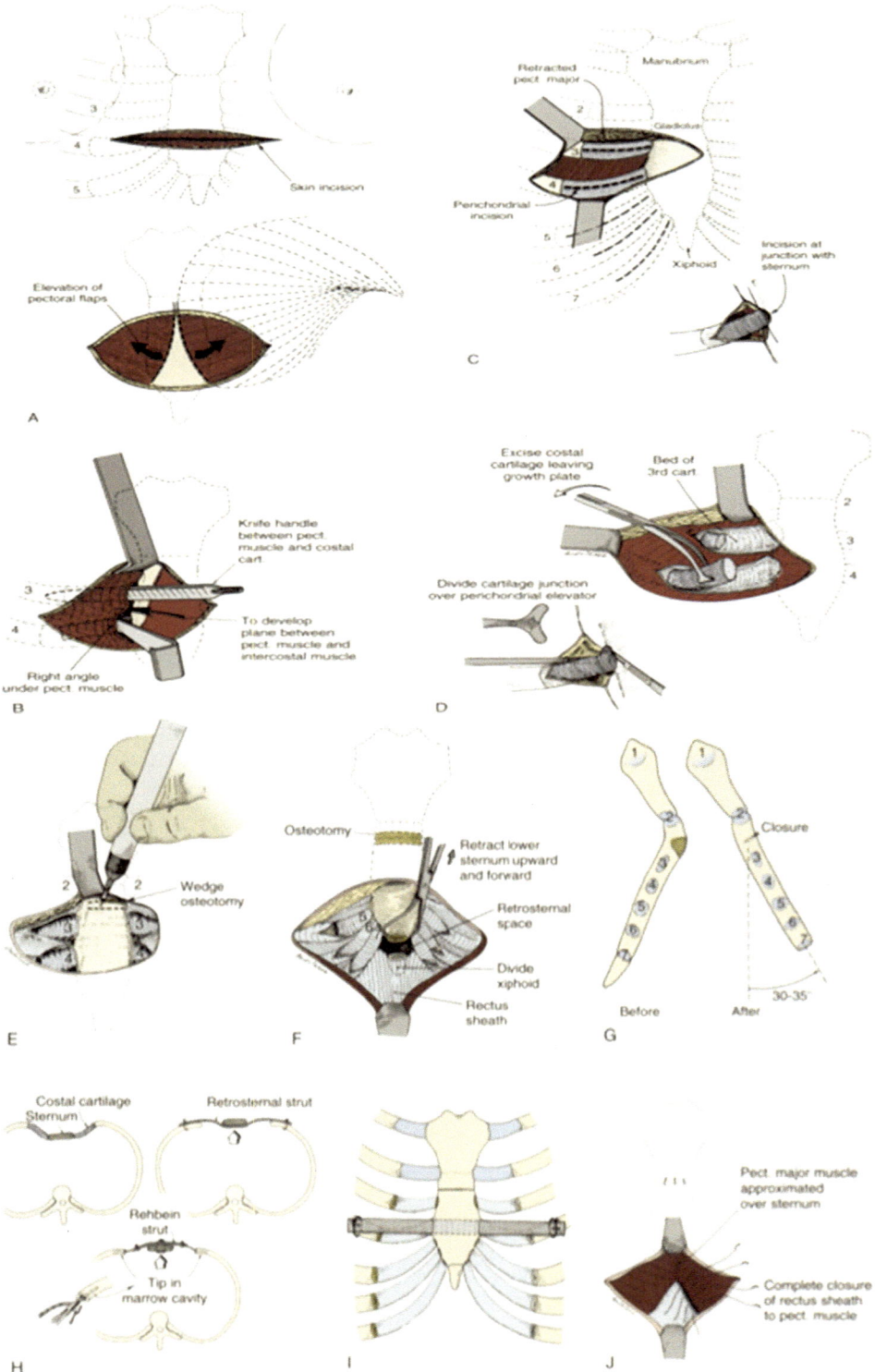

**Fig. 2.3** Ravitch repair

for repair used by most centers are subjective exercise intolerance, abnormal pulmonary function testing, abnormal echocardiogram, exercise-induced asthma, body image issues, and a Haller index > 3.25.

## Nonoperative Management

### Exercise Programs

The large majority of patients who present to referral centers are diagnosed with mild or moderate deformities and do not meet criteria for surgical intervention. These patients are typically started on exercise and posture programs. This strategy is designed to strengthen cardiopulmonary function and improve posture to allow for increased chest wall expansion as the classic pectus posture can contribute to progression of the deformity. Daily breathing and posture exercises are prescribed and patients are encouraged to participate in aerobic activities and team sports to avoid a sedentary lifestyle, which can worsen symptoms. These patients are reevaluated annually to monitor compliance and progression [41].

### Sternal Suction Device

Several case series in Europe using sternal suction devices applied to the anterior chest wall have reported success in managing patients with mild deformities. The device is used daily for 12–15 months and preliminary studies demonstrate correction of the sternal depression at approximately 1 cm per month. Long-term outcomes with the device, however, are still pending [42–45].

## Operative Management

### Open Repair (Modified Ravitch Repair)

The open approach requires a transverse inframammary skin incision at the level of the deepest portion of the sternal defect. Skin and muscle flaps are raised elevating the pectoralis muscles to expose the entire length of the affected portion of the sternum and bilateral costal cartilages. Subperichondrial resection of all abnormal costal cartilages is performed from the union with the rib laterally to the chondrosternal junction medially via an incision along the anterior surface of the perichondrium and dissection in the avascular plane between the costal cartilage and the surrounding perichondrium. Care must be taken to preserve the perichondrium to avoid devascularization. The xiphoid is then mobilized creating a substernal plane sweeping the pleura and pericardium off their attachments to the posterior sternum. A wedge osteotomy is created to neutralize the posterior depression of the sternum. A retrosternal bar or cartilage tripods are inserted to support the sternum. The incision is then closed and retrosternal and subcutaneous chest drains are typically left in place and removed 2–3 days later [34, 46].

Further modifications to the Ravitch procedure have been described and performed at select centers. The Leonard modification uses a retrosternal wire fixated to an external brace worn for 3 months as sternal support rather than a retrosternal bar [47] and the Robicsek modification stabilizes the sternum using Marlex mesh fixed to the cartilage remnants [48] (Fig. 2.3).

### Nuss Procedure

The minimally invasive approach described by Nuss involves surgically placing a convex steel bar underneath the sternum through small bilateral incisions. The bar is kept in place for 2–4 years allowing the sternum to reposition and remodel the deformed cartilage and rotate into a neutral position prior to removal. The original Nuss procedure has since been modified to use thoracoscopic guidance to visualize dissection of the transthoracic retrosternal plane for bar placement and to fixate the support bar in place with pericostal suturing to minimize postoperative displacement [34]. Bilateral thoracoscopic guidance or a subxiphoid incision can also help guide placement of the bar. The Nuss Procedure

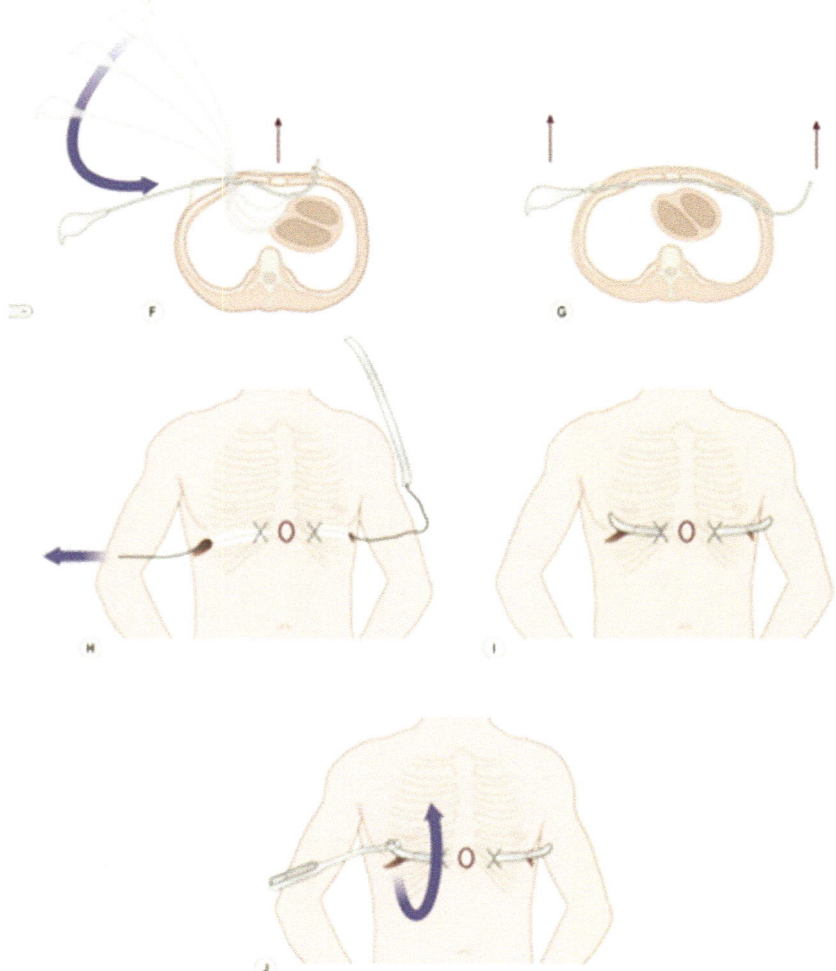

**Fig. 2.4** Nuss repair

has become the initial procedure of choice for many pediatric surgeons who believe it to be less radical with better cosmetic results [49–52] (Fig. 2.4).

## Complications

Pectus excavatum repair is generally well tolerated by patients with low rates of morbidity and mortality. A recent systematic review performed by Johnson et al. demonstrated that complication rates are similar for both procedures; however, to date, there is yet to be a randomized control trial looking at outcome differences between the two surgical approaches. Thus, the choice of operative procedure is primarily dependent on patient, surgeon, and institutional preference [15, 53–55].

The most common complications following pectus repair are bar-related events after the Nuss procedure such as displacement requiring reoperation (5.7–12 %) and pneumothorax (2–3.5 %). Wound infections (1.4–2.2 %) and pulmonary complications (2 %) such as effusions, atelectasis, and pneumonias also can occur but at less frequent rates. A recent analysis of patients undergoing the Nuss procedure using the NSQIP-P database reported a morbidity rate of

3.8 %, readmission rate of 3.8 %, and surgical site infection rate of 0.4 % [51, 52, 55–58]. Other rare but notable complications following the Nuss procedure include case reports of fatal or near-fatal hemorrhage during bar removal due to laceration of the pulmonary vessel or erosion into the sternum or aorta, or from bar rotation and erosion into the internal mammary artery [59–63]. Cases of cardiac tamponade and shock due to strut rotation and erosion to the aorta, bilateral sternoclavicular dislocation, and thoracic outlet obstruction have also been reported [62, 64, 65].

A rare but dreaded complication of the open pectus excavatum repair is acquired Jeune Syndrome (asphyxiating thoracic chondrodystrophy). In 1996, Haller et al. [66] first described 12 children who presented with severe restrictive cardiopulmonary symptoms due to a permanent impairment of normal chest wall growth after undergoing a Ravitch repair. The etiology is not completely clear; however, it is hypothesized that this life-threatening complication is the result of extensive and overzealous resection of the deformed cartilage with possible devascularization of the ossification center of the sternum. Early age of initial repair (less than 4 years old) may also increase the risk of this complication. Pulmonary function tests in these patients demonstrate a marked decreased FVC of 30–50 % and FEV1 of 30–60 %. Treatment is complex and requires re-excision of all substernal cartilage and using rib grafts or substernal support systems to reexpand the compressed chest cavity [67, 68].

## Outcomes

The majority of patients report excellent patient satisfaction regardless of operative approach type. The psychological benefits have long been well documented in the literature [69]. A large multicenter trial by Kelly et al. [70] demonstrated significant improvements in patient's body image difficulties and subjective limitations in physical activity after pectus repair. Ninety-seven percent of patients were satisfied with the postoperative cosmetic results.

Historically, recurrence rates prior to the introduction of the Nuss procedure ranged from 2 to 37 % [52]. More recent studies quote rates between 1.4 and 8.5 % [71, 72]. It was previously thought that the incidence of recurrence is higher in patients who are younger with connective tissue disorders or those who have had previous repairs [73]. However, Sacco-Casamassima et al. [71] did not find any significant patient or procedural factor predictive of recurrence in their series of 85 patients with recurrent pectus excavatum.

## Other Operative Interventions

### Prosthetic Inserts

Small case series in Europe and South America [74–77] have been reported treating pectus patients who present with solely cosmetic issues with custom-made silicone prosthetic implants to improve the outward appearance of the chest without changing the sternal shape. The procedure is generally well tolerated with satisfactory cosmetic outcomes. The most common complication reported is seroma formation in up to 30 % of patients [77]; however, no long-term studies have been reported.

### Magnetic Mini-Mover Procedure (3MP)

The magnetic mini-mover procedure [78–80] was designed to use magnetic force to gradually remodel the pectus excavatum deformity. Rather than a large magnitude of force applied at once, a magnetic field is used to apply a small amount of force over an extended period of time. This persistent gentle force theoretically allows the sternum to remold slowly and avoids the significant pain associated with traditional surgical procedures. A disc magnet is inserted surgically through a small subxiphoid incision and secured onto the sternum. A custom-made orthotic brace houses an external magnet and is fitted to the patient's chest. Patients wear the brace from 18 to

24 months until the internal magnet is subsequently removed. The initial pilot study did not result in a significant change in Haller index in their ten patients at 1 year of follow up, but there was a trend towards improvement in a subset of younger patients under 14. Further analysis demonstrated that the device proved to be safe and cost efficient. Currently, the magnetic minimover is in phase 3 multicenter trials.

# References

1. Jaroszewski D, et al. Current management of pectus excavatum: a review and update of therapy and treatment recommendations. J Am Board Fam Med. 2010;23(2):230–9.
2. Kelly Jr RE, et al. Pectus excavatum in a 112-year autopsy series: anatomic findings and the effect on survival. J Pediatr Surg. 2005;40(8):1275–8.
3. Fonkalsrud EW. Current management of pectus excavatum. World J Surg. 2003;27(5):502–8.
4. Brochhausen C, et al. Pectus excavatum: history, hypotheses and treatment options. Interact Cardiovasc Thorac Surg. 2012;14(6):801–6.
5. Bauhinus J. Sterni cum costis ad interna reflexis nativa spirandi difficultatis causa, in Grafenberg: Observationum rarum, novarum, admirabilium et monstruosorum 1609. In: Ioannis Schenckii a Grafenberg. Frankfurt: Tomus I Librum II. p. 507–8.
6. Toth GA, Buda BL. Funnel Chest (pectus excavatum) in 10-16th century fossil material. J Paleontol. 2001;13(2):63–6.
7. Kelly Jr RE. Pectus excavatum: historical background, clinical picture, preoperative evaluation and criteria for operation. Semin Pediatr Surg. 2008;17(3):181–93.
8. Meyer L. Zur chirurgischen Behandlung der angeborenen Trichterbrust. Berl Klin Wschr. 1911;48:1563–6.
9. Sauerbruch F. Operative Beseitigung der angeborenen Trichterbrust. Dtsch Z Chir. 1931;234(1):760–4.
10. Ravitch MM. The operative treatment of pectus excavatum. Ann Surg. 1949;129(4):429–44.
11. Wada J, et al. Results of 271 funnel chest operations. Ann Thorac Surg. 1970;10(6):526–32.
12. Nuss D, et al. A 10-year review of a minimally invasive technique for the correction of pectus excavatum. J Pediatr Surg. 1998;33(4):545–52.
13. Hansen JT, Netter FH. Netter's clinical anatomy. 3rd ed. Philadelphia: Saunders/Elsevier; 2014. xxii, p. 546.
14. Leung AK, Hoo JJ. Familial congenital funnel chest. Am J Med Genet. 1987;26(4):887–90.
15. Kelly Jr RE, et al. Prospective multicenter study of surgical correction of pectus excavatum: design, peri-operative complications, pain, and baseline pulmonary function facilitated by internet-based data collection. J Am Coll Surg. 2007;205(2):205–16.
16. Fonkalsrud EW, Dunn JC, Atkinson JB. Repair of pectus excavatum deformities: 30 years of experience with 375 patients. Ann Surg. 2000;231(3):443–8.
17. Stacey MW, et al. Variable number of tandem repeat polymorphisms (VNTRs) in the ACAN gene associated with pectus excavatum. Clin Genet. 2010;78(5):502–4.
18. Creswick HA, et al. Family study of the inheritance of pectus excavatum. J Pediatr Surg. 2006;41(10):1699–703.
19. Kotzot D, Schwabegger AH. Etiology of chest wall deformities—a genetic review for the treating physician. J Pediatr Surg. 2009;44(10):2004–11.
20. Cobben JM, Oostra RJ, van Dijk FS. Pectus excavatum and carinatum. Eur J Med Genet. 2014;57(8):414–7.
21. Colombani PM. Preoperative assessment of chest wall deformities. Semin Thorac Cardiovasc Surg. 2009;21(1):58–63.
22. Nakaoka T, et al. Does overgrowth of costal cartilage cause pectus excavatum? A study on the lengths of ribs and costal cartilages in asymmetric patients. J Pediatr Surg. 2009;44(7):1333–6.
23. Geisbe H, et al. [88. Biochemical, morphological and physical as well as animal experimental studies on the pathogenesis of funnel chest]. Langenbecks Arch Chir. 1967;319:536–41.
24. Rupprecht H, et al. Pathogenesis of chest wall abnormalities—electron microscopy studies and trace element analysis of rib cartilage. Z Kinderchir. 1987;42(4):228–9.
25. Fokin AA, et al. Anatomical, histologic, and genetic characteristics of congenital chest wall deformities. Semin Thorac Cardiovasc Surg. 2009;21(1):44–57.
26. Feng J, et al. The biomechanical, morphologic, and histochemical properties of the costal cartilages in children with pectus excavatum. J Pediatr Surg. 2001;36(12):1770–6.
27. Waters P, et al. Scoliosis in children with pectus excavatum and pectus carinatum. J Pediatr Orthop. 1989;9(5):551–6.
28. Hong JY, et al. Correlations of adolescent idiopathic scoliosis and pectus excavatum. J Pediatr Orthop. 2011;31(8):870–4.
29. Wang Y, et al. Mechanical factors play an important role in pectus excavatum with thoracic scoliosis. J Cardiothorac Surg. 2012;7:118.
30. Kelly Jr RE, Shamberger RC. Chapter 62—congenital chest wall deformities. In: Coran AG, editor. Pediatric surgery. 7th ed. Philadelphia: Mosby; 2012. p. 779–808.
31. Koumbourlis AC, Stolar CJ. Lung growth and function in children and adolescents with idiopathic pectus excavatum. Pediatr Pulmonol. 2004;38(4):339–43.
32. Kelly Jr RE, et al. Multicenter study of pectus excavatum, final report: complications, static/exercise pulmonary function, and anatomic outcomes. J Am Coll Surg. 2013;217(6):1080–9.

33. Malek MH, et al. Pulmonary function following surgical repair of pectus excavatum: a meta-analysis. Eur J Cardiothorac Surg. 2006;30(4):637–43.

34. Franz F, Goretsky M, Shamberger R. Pectus excavatum. In: Ziegler M et al., editors. Operative pediatric surgery. 2nd ed. New York: McGraw-Hill; 2014.

35. Shamberger RC, Welch KJ, Sanders SP. Mitral valve prolapse associated with pectus excavatum. J Pediatr. 1987;111(3):404–7.

36. Coln E, Carrasco J, Coln D. Demonstrating relief of cardiac compression with the Nuss minimally invasive repair for pectus excavatum. J Pediatr Surg. 2006;41(4):683–6. Discussion 683–6.

37. Malek MH, et al. Cardiovascular function following surgical repair of pectus excavatum: a metaanalysis. Chest. 2006;130(2):506–16.

38. Guntheroth WG, Spiers PS. Cardiac function before and after surgery for pectus excavatum. Am J Cardiol. 2007;99(12):1762–4.

39. Mueller C, Saint-Vil D, Bouchard S. Chest x-ray as a primary modality for preoperative imaging of pectus excavatum. J Pediatr Surg. 2008;43(1):71–3.

40. Haller Jr JA, Kramer SS, Lietman SA. Use of CT scans in selection of patients for pectus excavatum surgery: a preliminary report. J Pediatr Surg. 1987;22(10):904–6.

41. Nuss D, Kelly Jr RE. Minimally invasive surgical correction of chest wall deformities in children (Nuss procedure). Adv Pediatr. 2008;55:395–410.

42. Haecker FM, Mayr J. The vacuum bell for treatment of pectus excavatum: an alternative to surgical correction? Eur J Cardiothorac Surg. 2006;29(4):557–61.

43. Schier F, Bahr M, Klobe E. The vacuum chest wall lifter: an innovative, nonsurgical addition to the management of pectus excavatum. J Pediatr Surg. 2005;40(3):496–500.

44. Haecker FM. The vacuum bell for conservative treatment of pectus excavatum: the Basle experience. Pediatr Surg Int. 2011;27(6):623–7.

45. Lopez M, et al. Preliminary study of efficacy of cup suction in the correction of typical pectus excavatum. J Pediatr Surg. 2015;51(1):183–7.

46. Sultan I, Yang S. Congenital chest wall anomalies. In: Yuh DD, editor. Johns Hopkins textbook of cardiothoracic surgery. 2nd ed. New York: McGraw-Hill; 2014.

47. Antonoff MB, et al. When patients choose: comparison of Nuss, Ravitch, and Leonard procedures for primary repair of pectus excavatum. J Pediatr Surg. 2009;44(6):1113–9.

48. Robicsek F, Watts LT, Fokin AA. Surgical repair of pectus excavatum and carinatum. Semin Thorac Cardiovasc Surg. 2009;21(1):64–75.

49. Hebra A, et al. Outcome analysis of minimally invasive repair of pectus excavatum: review of 251 cases. J Pediatr Surg. 2000;35(2):252–7. Discussion 257–8.

50. Croitoru DP, et al. Experience and modification update for the minimally invasive Nuss technique for pectus excavatum repair in 303 patients. J Pediatr Surg. 2002;37(3):437–45.

51. Sacco-Casamassima MG, et al. Minimally invasive repair of pectus excavatum: analyzing contemporary practice in 50 ACS NSQIP-pediatric institutions. Pediatr Surg Int. 2015;31(5):493–9.

52. Kelly RE, et al. Twenty-one years of experience with minimally invasive repair of pectus excavatum by the Nuss procedure in 1215 patients. Ann Surg. 2010;252(6):1072–81.

53. de Oliveira Carvalho PE, et al. Surgical interventions for treating pectus excavatum. Cochrane Database Syst Rev. 2014;10:CD008889.

54. Johnson WR, Fedor D, Singhal S. Systematic review of surgical treatment techniques for adult and pediatric patients with pectus excavatum. J Cardiothorac Surg. 2014;9:25.

55. Nasr A, Fecteau A, Wales PW. Comparison of the Nuss and the Ravitch procedure for pectus excavatum repair: a meta-analysis. J Pediatr Surg. 2010;45(5):880–6.

56. Protopapas AD, Athanasiou T. Peri-operative data on the Nuss procedure in children with pectus excavatum: independent survey of the first 20 years' data. J Cardiothorac Surg. 2008;3:40.

57. Davis JT, Weinstein S. Repair of the pectus deformity: results of the Ravitch approach in the current era. Ann Thorac Surg. 2004;78(2):421–6.

58. Fonkalsrud EW, et al. Comparison of minimally invasive and modified Ravitch pectus excavatum repair. J Pediatr Surg. 2002;37(3):413–7.

59. Adam LA, Meehan JJ. Erosion of the Nuss bar into the internal mammary artery 4 months after minimally invasive repair of pectus excavatum. J Pediatr Surg. 2008;43(2):394–7.

60. Hoel TN, Rein KA, Svennevig JL. A life-threatening complication of the Nuss procedure for pectus excavatum. Ann Thorac Surg. 2006;81(1):370–2.

61. Jemielity M, et al. Life-threatening aortic hemorrhage during pectus bar removal. Ann Thorac Surg. 2011;91(2):593–5.

62. Leonhardt J, et al. Complications of the minimally invasive repair of pectus excavatum. J Pediatr Surg. 2005;40(11):e7–9.

63. Notrica DM, et al. Life-threatening hemorrhage during removal of a Nuss bar associated with sternal erosion. Ann Thorac Surg. 2014;98(3):1104–6.

64. Kilic B, et al. Vascular thoracic outlet syndrome developed after minimally invasive repair of pectus excavatum. Eur J Cardiothorac Surg. 2013;44(3):567–9.

65. Lee SH, Ryu SM, Cho SJ. Thoracic outlet syndrome after the Nuss procedure for the correction of extreme pectus excavatum. Ann Thorac Surg. 2011;91(6):1975–7.

66. Haller Jr JA, et al. Chest wall constriction after too extensive and too early operations for pectus excavatum. Ann Thorac Surg. 1996;61(6):1618–25.

67. Sacco Casamassima MG, et al. Operative management of acquired Jeune's syndrome. J Pediatr Surg. 2014;49(1):55–60. Discussion 60.

68. Phillips JD, van Aalst JA. Jeune's syndrome (asphyxiating thoracic dystrophy): congenital and acquired. Semin Pediatr Surg. 2008;17(3):167–72.
69. Einsiedel E, Clausner A. Funnel chest. Psychological and psychosomatic aspects in children, youngsters, and young adults. J Cardiovasc Surg (Torino). 1999;40(5):733–6.
70. Kelly Jr RE, et al. Surgical repair of pectus excavatum markedly improves body image and perceived ability for physical activity: multicenter study. Pediatrics. 2008;122(6):1218–22.
71. Sacco Casamassima MG, et al. Contemporary management of recurrent pectus excavatum. J Pediatr Surg. 2015;50(10):1726–33.
72. Redlinger Jr RE, et al. One hundred patients with recurrent pectus excavatum repaired via the minimally invasive Nuss technique—effective in most regardless of initial operative approach. J Pediatr Surg. 2011;46(6):1177–81.
73. Colombani PM. Recurrent chest wall anomalies. Semin Pediatr Surg. 2003;12(2):94–9.
74. Anger J, Alcalde RF, de Campos JR. The use of soft silicone solid implant molded intraoperatively for pectus excavatum surgical repair. Einstein (Sao Paulo). 2014;12(2):186–90.
75. Soccorso G, Parikh DH, Worrollo S. Customized silicone implant for the correction of acquired and congenital chest wall deformities: a valuable option with pectus excavatum. J Pediatr Surg. 2015;50(7):1232–5.
76. Wechselberger G, et al. Silicone implant correction of pectus excavatum. Ann Plast Surg. 2001;47(5):489–93.
77. Snel BJ, et al. Pectus excavatum reconstruction with silicone implants: long-term results and a review of the english-language literature. Ann Plast Surg. 2009;62(2):205–9.
78. Harrison MR, et al. Magnetic mini-mover procedure for pectus excavatum II: initial findings of a Food and Drug Administration-sponsored trial. J Pediatr Surg. 2010;45(1):185–91. Discussion 191–2.
79. Harrison MR, et al. Magnetic Mini-Mover Procedure for pectus excavatum: I. Development, design, and simulations for feasibility and safety. J Pediatr Surg. 2007;42(1):81–5. Discussion 85–6.
80. Harrison MR, et al. Magnetic mini-mover procedure for pectus excavatum III: safety and efficacy in a Food and Drug Administration-sponsored clinical trial. J Pediatr Surg. 2012;47(1):154–9.

# Magnetic Mini-Mover Procedure for Pectus Excavatum

Claire Graves and Shinjiro Hirose

The most common procedures for the repair of pectus excavatum, the Nuss and the Ravitch, correct the chest wall in a single procedure, forcing the sternum forward with extensive manipulation under general anesthesia. These procedures cause significant pain and can require lengthy hospitalization with extended recovery. The magnetic mini-mover procedure (3MP) for pectus excavatum was developed as an alternative to these procedures. Inspired by orthodontic braces and bracing for pectus carinatum, the procedure applies a small amount of force over a long period of time to achieve chest wall correction. The 3MP uses a magnetic field to apply controlled outward force on the sternum, gradually re-forming the chest wall cartilage over time without major surgery or hospitalization. Moreover, once a good correction has been achieved, the position of the sternum can be adjusted or held in place while cartilage remodeling completes with intermittent bracing, much like a nightly retainer holds the teeth in place after braces have been removed.

C. Graves
Department of Surgery, Columbia University,
177 Fort Washington Ave, New York,
NY 10032, USA

S. Hirose, M.D. (✉)
Division of Pediatric General, Thoracic, and Fetal
Surgery, UC Davis Medical Center, Shriners
Hospitals for Children—Northern California,
2425 Stockton Blvd, Sacramento, CA, USA
e-mail: shirose@ucdavis.edu

## 3MP Device

The 3MP device consists of two parts: an internal magnet, which is implanted on the sternum, and an external magnet, which is integrated into a custom-fitted anterior chest wall brace (Fig. 3.1). The attraction between the internal and external magnets produces an outward force on the sternum. The device applies a steady, sustained force on the malformed costal cartilages, slowly remodeling the chest wall and correcting the deformity.

The internal, implanted magnet (Magnimplant) consists of 1½-in. diameter, 3/16-in. thick neodymium–iron–boron magnet backed by a 1/16-in. ferromagnetic plate (to focus the magnetic field in the direction of the brace), fully encased in a low-profile titanium shell (Fig. 3.2a). The device is positioned on the front of the sternum and secured to a titanium disk back plate on the posterior sternum. In the initial design, the anterior magnet casing included a threaded post on the posterior surface, which was inserted through a hole in the depressed portion of the sternum and screwed securely into a threaded stem on a titanium disk back plate. When treatment is completed, the device is removed in an outpatient procedure.

The external device (Magnatract) is a custom-made orthotic device made of polypropylene that is molded to each patient's chest wall (Fig. 3.2b).

© Springer International Publishing Switzerland 2017
G.W. Raff, S. Hirose (eds.), *Surgery for Chest Wall Deformities*,
DOI 10.1007/978-3-319-43926-6_3

**Fig. 3.1** Axial diagram of magnetic mini-mover procedure (3MP)

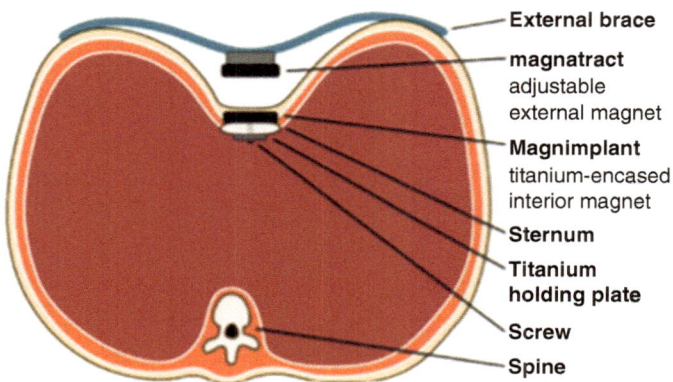

External brace

**magnatract** adjustable external magnet

**Magnimplant** titanium-encased interior magnet

**Sternum**

**Titanium holding plate**

**Screw**

**Spine**

**A**
Anterior plate containing magnet

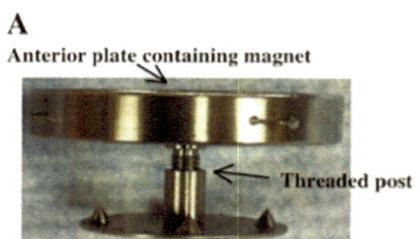

Threaded post

**B**

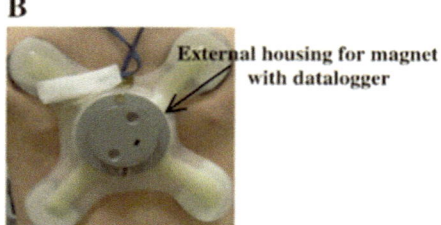

External housing for magnet with datalogger

**Fig. 3.2** 3MP device. (**a**) The Magnimplant consists of a neodymium–iron–boron rare-earth disc magnet (1.5 in. diameter × 0.1875 in. thick) and a ferromagnetic focusing plate encapsulated in a low-profile titanium shell that is positioned on the front of the sternum and is secured to the sternum by screwing it into the threaded stem of a tita-nium disk back plate. (**b**) The Magnatract is a custom-made, external orthotic brace with a housing unit for a second rare-earth magnet. The brace is held in place using the attractive force between the coupled internal and external magnets, and the force exerted on the sternum is adjustable

The Magnatract houses a second rare earth magnet that is held onto the patient's chest wall by its attraction to the implanted magnet. The position of the magnet within the brace is adjustable, so that the strength of the magnetic force can be regulated, allowing patient-specific alterations in force and orientation. The external device also includes sensors, which measure and record the temperature and the force generated when the magnet is exposed to the magnetic implant. This sensor is wired to a custom-designed microprocessor and data logger, which records the force and temperature every 10 min. Using these data, the patient and clinician can track how long the brace is worn and how much force the magnets are exerting.

## Development and Preclinical Testing

To demonstrate that the 3MP could apply enough force to reform the costal cartilages, the device was implanted in human skeletons to test the variation of force produced by attraction of the coupled magnets at various distances. The force generated on the internal magnet (and therefore the sternum) is 4.45 kg when the magnets are 1 cm apart. As the external magnet is adjusted further away, the outward force decreases (Fig. 3.3). The force necessary to move the chest wall 1 cm in an awake child is approximately 2.5–5.0 kg, varying with age and sex [1]. In contrast to traditional corrective procedures, which

**Fig. 3.3** Measurements of the strength and force generated by various distances of internal and external magnets

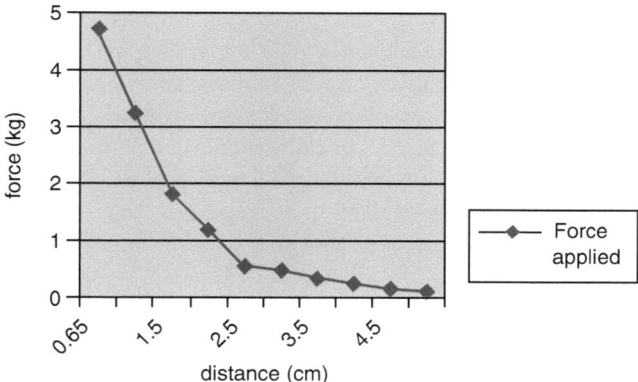

must move the chest wall a large distance at a single time and thus require a large amount of force (up to 23.4 kg), the 3MP must only apply enough force to stimulate the reformation of the abnormal cartilages. This stimulus can then be continuously applied over a period of months. The outward force on the sternum generated by the two-magnet system, 4.45 kg when the magnets are 1 cm apart, is in the range required to move the sternum 1 cm in an awake child and therefore is in a range capable of producing a gradual remodeling of the chest wall.

A significant consideration during development of the device was the safety of long-term exposure to magnetic fields from an implanted magnet, especially one placed so near the heart. To determine the magnetic field strength at the surface of the heart generated by the device, a magnetic field map was drawn with the magnets at varying distances from 1 to 10 cm apart. When the magnets were 1 cm apart, the maximum field strength reaching the undersurface of the sternum was 0.04 T. From studies investigating the risk of magnetic resonance imaging on human safety, it is accepted that there is no detectable effect on cardiac performance or hemodynamics from exposure of magnetic fields up to 1.5 T [2, 3]. Moreover, an interesting large animal model exists in the prevention of *Bovine Hardware disease* with "cow magnets." These magnets are placed in one of the bovine stomachs to collect ingested wires, nails, and other metal that would otherwise cause trauma or obstruction more distally in the GI tract. The magnets, of a similar

strength and at a similar distance from the heart as the 3MP, remain in place for the animal's entire life with no ill effect [4].

Another early safety concern was whether the magnetic field generated by the device could pose a risk to others in close contact with the patient, or interfere with external devices. To decrease this risk, the Magnatract brace was covered with a thin ferromagnetic shield to decrease the magnetic field outward from the brace. Using the shield, the highest field strength at the outer surface of the orthosis decreased from 150 to 10 G [5].

## Phase I Clinical Trial

### Study Design

Following preclinical testing, we obtained an Investigational Device Exemption (G050196/A002) to proceed with trial in patients. Funded by a Food and Drug Administration (FDA) Office of Orphan Products grant (R01FD003341), a first-in-human trial was conducted to test the safety and proof of concept of the procedure. Ten otherwise healthy patients between 8 and 14 years of age with a pectus severity index greater than 3.5 were enrolled in the single-institution pilot study. After implantation of the Magnimplant device, patients wore their custom-fitted Magnatract external brace for the 18-month duration of the trial. Patients were followed with monthly wound checks and chest X-rays to monitor for skin changes and device integrity, respectively, and the pectus severity index (PSI) was recalculated over the course of treatment. Preoperative and post-implant removal chest CT scans were obtained to assess overall improvement in PSI. Electrocardiograms (EKGs) were obtained pre-implant, 1-month post-implant, and 1-month post-explant to monitor for any effect on cardiac electrical function.

## Safety

Seven boys and three girls with mean age 12.7 (range 8–14) years participated in the pilot trial. Patient data are summarized in Table 3.1. From sensor data, the average brace wear time was 16 h per day and generally increased over the course of the study. None of the patients developed EKG changes or had any clinical signs of cardiac effects. There were no incidents of permanent skin damage or discoloration from wearing the external orthotic device. One patient experienced some mild skin erythema, but this resolved with brace reconfiguration. There were no infections from device implantation or chronic use, but three patients had a postoperative wound infection following implant removal, including one patient who

required hospital admission for intravenous antibiotics and wound exploration for possible osteomyelitis, which proved negative. One patient developed a pericardial effusion 16 months after implantation, which required urgent pericardiocentesis. On extensive work-up, no evidence on imaging, echocardiogram, blood, or skin tests demonstrated an association with the implanted magnet, and it was left in place. No recurrent effusion developed, and the evaluating consultants concluded the effusion was likely viral in origin.

In three patients, a routine monthly X-ray demonstrated a device breakage at the weld point between the posterior plate and the threaded post. Patients were asymptomatic, and none of the devices had migrated, likely due to the fibrous capsule that develops around the device. All three of these devices were immediately removed with an outpatient procedure due to safety concerns. One subject was withdrawn from the study early due to this device failure, but elected to continue treatment (subject S0008, starred in Table 3.1). Three other outpatient reoperations were required. One procedure was to loosen an overtightened implant that was causing persistent pain, and two procedures were to reattach or replace a device that had uncoupled due to misalignment of the

**Table 3.1** Data of mean compliance per 24 h and pectus severity index pretreatment and posttreatment

| Subject | Age at implant, years | Sex | Total months in study | Mean compliance, % | Pectus severity index at enrollment | Final pectus severity index | Correction, % |
|---------|------|-----|------|------|------|------|------|
| S0001 | 14 | Male | 18 | 48.8 | 4.3 | 3.48 | 78.1 |
| S0002 | 14 | Male | 17 | 86.2 | 3.71 | 3.55 | 34.8 |
| S0003 | 14 | Female | 20 | 60.5 | 3.6 | 4.24 | −182.9 |
| S0004 | 12 | Female | 17 | 72.9 | 6.1 | 6.37 | −9.5 |
| S0005 | 11 | Male | 25 | 61.2 | 3.96 | 3.01 | 133.8 |
| S0006 | 8 | Female | 16 | 71.1 | 4.19 | 3.66 | 56.4 |
| S0007 | 12 | Male | 19 | 67.6 | 7.3 | 8.12 | −20.2 |
| S0008[a] | 14 | Male | 19 | 92 | 4.86 | 3.76 | 68.3 |
| S0009 | 14 | Male | 18 | 74.5 | 4.1 | 5 | −105.9 |
| S00010 | 14 | Male | 19 | 65.6 | 5.66 | 7.65 | −82.6 |

Achieved percentage of ideal correction is defined as $[(PSI_{pretreatment} - PSI_{current})/(PSI_{pretreatment} - PSI_{cutoff})] \times 100$, where $PSI_{cutoff} = 3.25$ (cutoff value that differentiates normal control from pectus excavatum patient population)
[a]S0008 was withdrawn from study and overall analysis because of the early device failure
*PSI* indicates pectus severity index

cross-threading between the two components during implantation. In total, six reoperations were undertaken in five patients.

## Proof of Concept

A surprising finding from the pilot study was the difficulty in reliably measuring pectus severity. Using pretreatment and posttreatment CT scans, no significant change in PSI was demonstrated. However, throughout the study, neither CT scans nor chest X-rays were reproducible from one exam to the next, largely due to variability in patient positioning and respiratory cycle, as well as scattering of the CT image by the implanted magnet. Moreover, all patients involved in the study were peripubertal. PSI is known to worsen during the rapid growth spurt of puberty in most patients, and there is no reliable control data on the degree of worsening with which to compare the 3MP patients. In other words, there is no way to know whether the 3MP prevented or lessened the expected worsening during the pubertal growth spurt. Greater improvement was seen in the patients who were in the early or midpubertal growth spurt than in patients nearing the end of the growth spurt. Subjectively, patients were "unsure" to "satisfied" with the degree of correction of their chest on posttreatment surveys, and seven of nine patients would recommend the treatment to someone else.

## Clinical Device Adaptations

Using the device in clinical practice for the first time sparked significant adaptations of the device and procedure. First, the surgical procedure to place the Magnimplant evolved through the course of the ten patients. The device is designed to be placed through a 3-cm incision at the xiphoid–sternal junction. The xiphoid is separated from the lower sternum with electrocautery and blunt dissection, and a space is created in front of and behind the sternum to create a pocket for the implant. Creating a hole in the sternum for the joining of the magnet to the back plate was time

consuming and difficult with a drill, so we developed a punch anvil that quickly and effectively created the hole (Fig. 3.4a, b). However, blindly guiding the posterior plate through the small incision and into the correct location behind the sternal hole also proved challenging. To make this step much faster and simpler, we developed a flexible monofilament guidewire that was screwed into the back plate post and used to guide it into the proper position (Fig. 3.4c–e). The guidewire is unscrewed, and the anterior magnet is mated and screwed into the back plate to secure it onto the sternum. Operative time decreased from 105 to 30 min throughout the course of the trial as techniques and instruments evolved.

The external Magnatract device also evolved throughout the trial, as patient feedback at monthly visits facilitated iterative reengineering and modifications. From bench top testing, we knew that the optimal configuration to maximize magnetic force was an N55 NdFeB rare-earth magnet encased in a steel focusing cup. The external magnet needs to be as close as possible to the sternal magnet without touching the skin to maximize outward pull. Our initial 3-in. diameter housing was unable to lie close to the chest wall in girls with developing breasts, so we reduced the casing to 1.5- and 2-in. diameter. We also adapted the casing to allow patients to adjust the force of the magnetic pull. The magnet and housing are threaded such that the patient can twist the external magnet in a "nut" on the brace in order to move it closer or father from the chest wall and internal magnet (Fig. 3.5). Thus, if the patient feels discomfort from too much pull, the magnet could be adjusted further from the chest wall to quickly decrease magnetic force.

## Cost Effectiveness

We compared patient care costs, including surgical, anesthesia, and hospital costs, for study patients with those of patients who underwent either the Nuss or Ravitch procedure at our institution during the same period. Excluding additional costs associated with tests or procedures unique to the study protocol (e.g. follow-up CT scans, chest

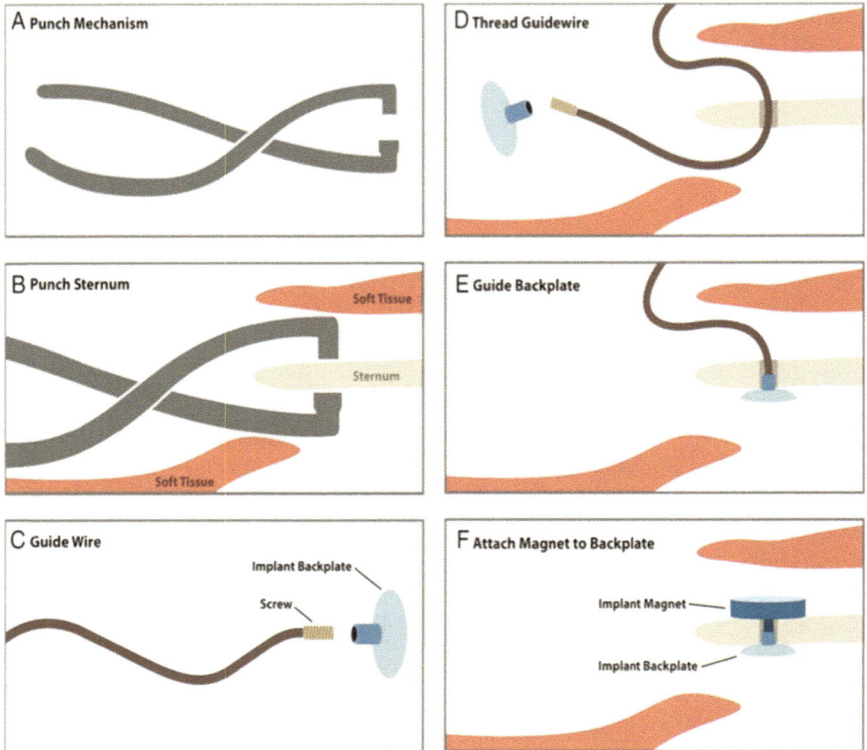

**Fig. 3.4** (**a**) Sternal punch device. (**b**) Sternal punch engaged with deepest point of sternal defect through subxiphoid incision. (**c**) Guide wire with posterior plate of implant. (**d**) Guide wire through sternal hole coupling with posterior plate. (**e**) Guide wire with posterior plate in place. (**f**) Magnimplant on sternum

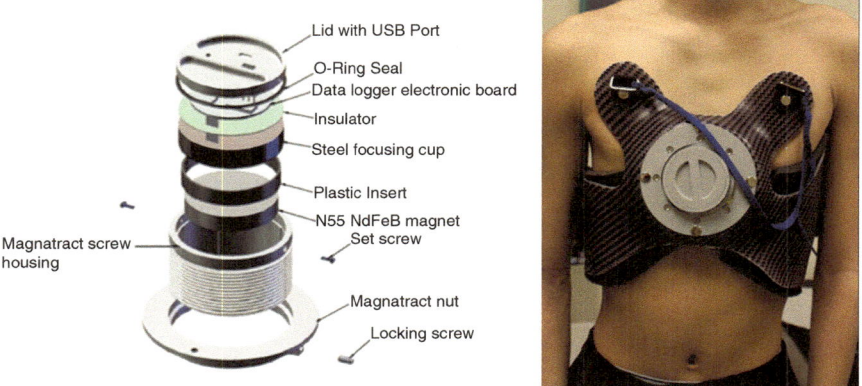

**Fig. 3.5** Magnatract device for adjustable housing of external magnet, which is then incorporated into custom-fitted chest wall brace

x-rays, and monthly clinic visits), which would not be standard of care the general population, the cost of 3MP was 58 % of the standard Nuss or Ravitch procedures at our institution during the same time period, $46,859 vs. $81,114 [6].

## Conclusions from Pilot Trial

The pilot study revealed no detectable ill effect on cardiac function, wound repair, or bone and cartilage stability from the magnet field or frequent force applied to the sternum. Significant progress in device design and procedural technique was made through the course of the study, which led to significantly easier and faster implantation, as well as more comfortable and effective external braces. The three mechanical failures at the weld of the internal posterior plate to its threaded post and the two cases of decoupling of the implant due to misalignment led to a redesign of the implant in order to eliminate these problems in the future.

Though quantitative evaluation of pectus excavatum severity proved difficult throughout the pilot trial, younger patients (ages 8–12 years) had dramatic initial improvement with the device, likely due to the increased compliance of the chest wall in this age group, whose costal cartilages are not yet ossified. The effect, however, can be lost when treatment is terminated prior to the pubertal growth spurt, as pectus deformities are known to increase in severity during this time. Patients who wore the brace for longer periods of time also had more rapid correction. Thus, the trial identified patients who would benefit most from the treatment and suggested that a longer duration of treatment than the proscribed 18 months may be more effective [7, 6].

## Phase II Clinical Trial

To implement the lessons learned from the initial pilot trial and supplement data from the initial pilot trial, a Phase II trial of 15 otherwise healthy patients with pectus excavatum is currently underway, funded by a grant from the FDA's Office of Orphan Products Development. The trial implements several important modifications from Phase I trial. First, the duration of treatment was extended by the FDA to 24 months (from the original 18 months). Second, the Magnimplant has been redesigned to eliminate the problematic threaded post coupling system. Instead, the titanium-encased anterior magnet is secured to the sternum with titanium cables that attach to a titanium back plate (Fig. 3.6). With this modification, dissection is

**Fig. 3.6** Redesigned Magnimplant for Phase II trial. The new design eliminates the threaded coupling system and welded components, which proved problematic in the pilot trial

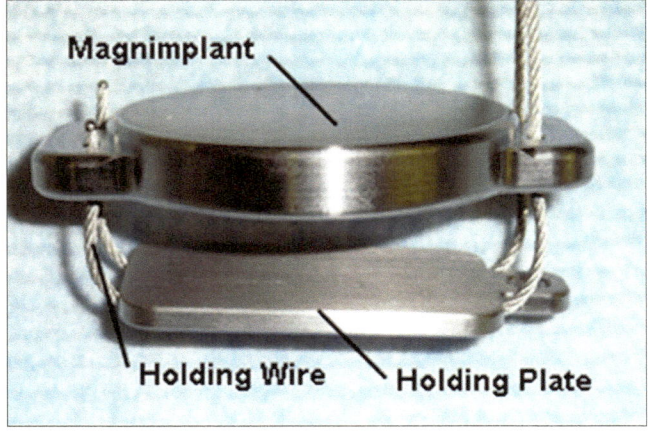

minimized and removal of the device is simplified. The external Magnatract device retained the functions that evolved throughout the first trial, including the screw mechanism for patient-adjustable magnet strength and sensors for recording frequency and duration of brace wear. Third, to further evaluate the role of bone age in the efficacy of the device, all patients received a wrist X-ray for bone age determination prior to treatment. This trial is currently in progress.

## Summary

In patients with pectus excavatum, the magnetic mini-mover procedure (3MP) is used to apply a gradual, sustained force on the sternum to slowly remodel the malformed costal cartilages. This approach allows chest wall correction without the significant pain and lengthy hospitalization associated with the Nuss and Ravitch procedures. We describe development, design, and preclinical simulations for feasibility and safety. A Phase I trial of ten patients demonstrated safety of device implantation and treatment. Results on efficacy were mixed, but were promising in younger, prepubertal patients with more compliant chest walls. The initial trial prompted modifications of technique as well as design revisions for both the implant and the external brace. A multicenter trial of 15 patients using the redesigned device is currently underway.

## References

1. Boia SE, Susan-Resigna R, Raicov PC, et al. Determination of the mechanical requirements for progressive correction system of pectus excavatum in children. J Laparoendosc Adv Surg Tech. 2005;15(5):478–81.
2. Chakeres DW, Kangarlu A, Boudaoulas H, et al. Effect of static magnetic field exposure of up to 8 Tesla on sequential human vital sign measurements. J Magn Reson Imaging. 2003;18(3):346–52.
3. Tenforde TS. Magnetically induced fields and currents in the circulatory system. Prog Biophys Mol Biol. 2005;87(2-3):279–88.
4. Kahn CM, Line S. The Merck veterinary manual. 9th ed. Hoboken: Wiley; 2005.
5. Harrison MR, Estefan-Ventura D, Fechter R, et al. Magnetic mini-mover procedure for pectus excavatum I: development, design, and simulations for feasibility and safety. J Pediatr Surg. 2007;42:81–5.
6. Harrison MR, Gonzales K, Bratton B, et al. Magnetic mini-mover procedure for pectus excavatum III: safety and efficacy in a Food and Drug Administration-sponsored trial. J Pediatr Surg. 2012;47:154–9.
7. Harrison MR, Curran PF, Jamshidi R, et al. Magnetic mini-mover procedure for pectus excavatum II: initial findings of a Food and Drug Administration-sponsored trial. J Pediatr Surg. 2010;45:185–91.

# Pectus Carinatum

## Yuen Julia Chen and Shinjiro Hirose

## Introduction

Pectus carinatum, "keel chest" or "pigeon chest," is a congenital chest wall disorder characterized by an anterior convex protrusion of the chest wall. The incidence of pectus carinatum is approximately 0.06 % of live births with a male predominance of 4:1 [1, 2]. It is approximately five to six times less common than pectus excavatum [3, 4] but is the second most common chest wall deformity seen in children [5].

The anatomical site and degree of displacement of the sternum in pectus carinatum falls along a spectrum and can be broadly divided into four categories [6]. The most frequent form is symmetrical chondrogladiolar which is characterized by a symmetrical anterior protrusion of the body of the sternum with protrusion of the lower costal cartilages [7]. This deformity is found in up to 95 % of children with pectus carinatum [8, 9]. The physical appearance has been likened to the anterior portion of the chest being pinched forward by a giant hand. Asymmetrical chondrogladiolar deformity is the next most common subtype with normal cartilage on one side and anterior displacement on the other. Mixed carinatum and excavatum deformities result in a carinatum deformity on one side and an excavatum deformity on the other. They are frequently associated with a component of sternal rotation. Finally, the least common subtype is the chondromanubrial deformity sometimes referred to as Currarino-Silverman Syndrome [10]. In chondromanubrial deformities, the upper portion of the chest including the manubrium and second and third costal cartilages protrude forward while the body of the sternum remains relatively depressed. The sternum is often foreshortened with absent segmentation or premature obliteration of the sternal sutures [10].

## Historical

Pectus carinatum has been a known condition since antiquity; Hippocrates described patients in which "the chest becomes sharp pointed, not broad, and becomes affected with difficulty in breathing and hoarseness" [9].

In 1952, Ravitch first reported repair of the carinatum defect in a patient with a chondromanubrial

Y.J. Chen, M.D.
Department of Surgery, Mount Sinai Medical Center, New York, NY, USA
e-mail: juchen@ucdavis.edu

S. Hirose, M.D. (✉)
Division of Pediatric General, Thoracic, and Fetal Surgery, UC Davis Medical Center, Shriners Hospitals for Children—Northern California, 2425 Stockton Blvd, Sacramento, CA, USA
e-mail: shirose@ucdavis.edu

© Springer International Publishing Switzerland 2017
G.W. Raff, S. Hirose (eds.), *Surgery for Chest Wall Deformities*,
DOI 10.1007/978-3-319-43926-6_4

deformity and cardiac symptoms [11] and subsequent successful repairs of two additional patients with chondrogladiolar deformities in 1960. In Ravitch's initial report he described the carinatum deformity as "an unusual sternal deformity with cardiac symptoms." His repair involved resecting the deformed costal cartilage in either one or two stages and placing sutures to shorten and posteriorly displace the perichondrium [12]. Around the same time, Lester described a more radical resection that included subperiosteal removal of not only the costal cartilage but also the corresponding portion of the sternum [13]. In 1963, Robicsek reported success using subperichondrial resection of costal cartilages, a transverse sternal osteotomy and resection of the protruding lower sternum to treat the defect [14].

## Pathophysiology

The etiology of pectus carinatum remains unknown. Up to 30 % of cases are associated with a family history suggestive of a strong genetic component [1]. There is also a strong association with scoliosis and other spinal deformities in up to 15 % of patients suggestive of a global connective tissue disorder [5, 15]. Pectus carinatum has also been linked to congenital heart disease, Marfan Syndrome, Noonan Syndrome, and other connective tissue disorders. The exact genetic link is yet to be identified; however, there are reports of mutations in type II collagen (COL2A1) associated with pectus carinatum [16].

Both pectus carinatum and excavatum are thought to be the result of disordered cartilage growth. Rapid growth in one plane displaces the sternum forward resulting in the carinatum defect while growth in the opposite plane leads to posterior displacement of the sternum resulting in the excavatum deformity [17]. Park et al. [18] used three-dimensional computed tomography (CT) to evaluate 26 patients with symmetric pectus carinatum and compared with matched control subjects. They concluded that the lengths of costal cartilages were significantly longer in patients with pectus carinatum supporting the theory that overgrowth at the costal cartilage contributes to the development of the carinatum defect.

## Presentation

Pectus carinatum rarely can present at birth; however, it typically progresses during childhood at periods of growth and becomes truly clinically apparent during the early teenage years. The chondromanubrial deformity, however, unlike the chondrogladiolar deformity, is more frequently noted at birth.

## Clinical Features

The diagnosis of pectus carinatum is one based on clinical findings. The most common presenting symptoms are body image issues and psychosocial concerns. Similar to patients who present with pectus excavatum, these body image issues should not be underrated as they have been associated with a dramatic reduction in quality of life [19] and warrants an aggressive evaluation. Those patients who do manifest physical symptoms report exertional dyspnea, exercise limitations, frequent respiratory infections, and chest discomfort or pain [3]. These respiratory symptoms may be the result of impaired ventilation from a fixed chest wall and increased residual lung volumes [4]. Of note, there is an association with congenital heart disease in patients with the chondromanubrial defect with a reported 18 % of children with identified sternal fusion anomalies presenting with documented congenital heart disease [20].

## Clinical Assessment

For most patients, pectus carinatum is easily diagnosed clinically. A thorough history and physical helps to guide the need for further testing, which is rarely indicated. If there are no features of a global disorder identified, then genetic studies are also not indicated. There is some literature supporting the use of routine CT scans for preoperative evaluation and planning [21]; however, others advocate for the use of plain film only [5]. Rarely, do patients require additional testing; however, those who present with cardiopulmonary symptoms may benefit from pulmonary function tests (PFTs) and a full cardiac workup.

## Management

Most patients who present with pectus carinatum are managed nonoperatively. The indications for surgical correction include pain, respiratory symptoms, ease of injury, psychosocial concerns related to body image, and failure of nonoperative techniques. Surgical repair is typically deferred until completion of puberty given the high chance of recurrence with those patients who undergo intervention prior to completion of the pubertal growth spurts [17].

## Operative Repair

Operative intervention on pectus carinatum is essentially the modified open Ravitch repair that is used for pectus excavatum repair. All abnormal cartilage is removed via subperichondrial resection allowing the sternum to return to a neutral position. The key to a successful repair of the

defect is identifying and removing all abnormal cartilages as any remaining abnormal cartilages represent sources of recurrence [1].

Various techniques have been described depending on the subtype of deformity involved. For patients who present with a chondrogladiolar deformity, a single or double osteotomy allows for the posterior plate of the sternum to be fractured and returned to a normal position. In mixed deformities, a wedge osteotomy on the anterior sternal plate is often required to correct the oblique position of the sternum. The closure of the osteotomy subsequently elevates and rotates the sternum into the correct position. In the chondromanubrial deformity, a wedge osteotomy is made in the anterior plate of the sternum where the point of maximal protrusion occurs. Upon closure, the lower sternum is brought anteriorly and the manubrium rotates posteriorly into a normal position (Fig. 4.1) [2]. Meshes and struts have been described as mechanisms of further sternal support if needed [9, 22]. Further modifications of the original technique

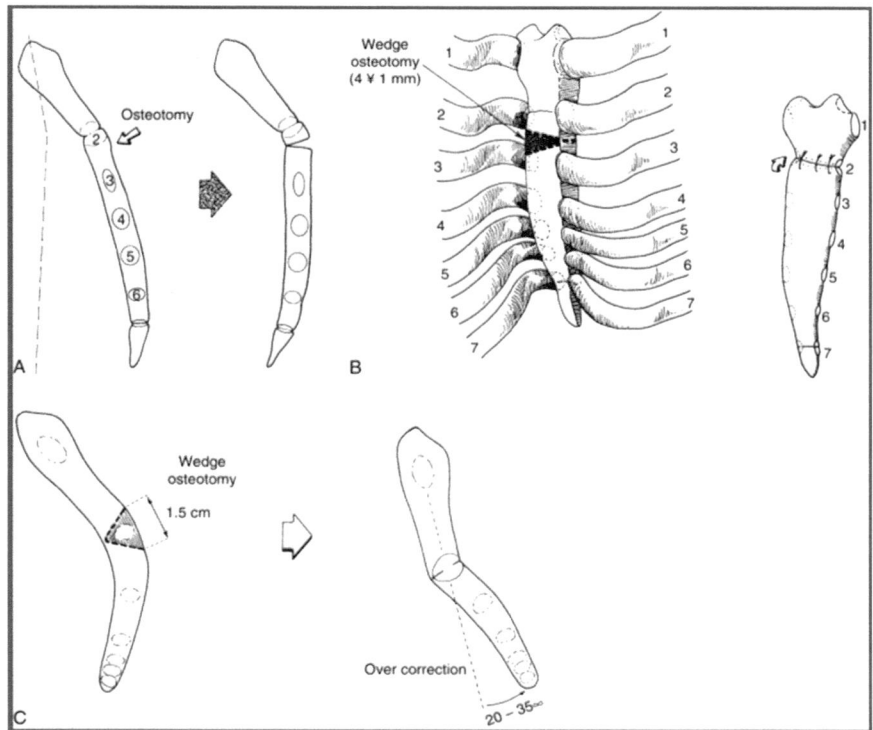

**Fig. 4.1** (**a**) Chondrogladiolar repair; (**b**) mixed deformity repair; (**c**) chondromanubrial repair (From Chondrogladiolar.) [2]

include reduced cartilage resection, less extensive dissections with sternal plating, and postoperative bracing [23, 24].

Outcomes following the modified Ravitch repair for pectus carinatum are fairly positive with high postoperative patient satisfaction rates [25] and minimal complications. Complications reported include seroma, wound infection, pleural effusions, pneumothorax, and local tissue necrosis [1, 26]. Recurrence rates are reported to be 1.8–5.5 % [23, 24, 27]. Most authors advocate for delaying repair until after puberty in order to reduce the rate of recurrence [28].

The first minimally invasive technique for pectus carinatum repair was described in 1997 by Kobayashi et al. using a subcutaneous endoscopic technique with multiple stab incisions to facilitate the cartilage resection [29]. Other techniques described in the literature include using subpectoral insufflation or thoracoscopic-assisted methods to assist with rib resection [30, 31]. These techniques involve novel minimally invasive methods of creating operative space to perform the rib resection; however, widespread use is yet to be adopted.

In 2009, Abramson et al. described a novel technique not requiring cartilage resection to treat pectus carinatum in which a curved steel bar is inserted subcutaneously and fixed to the lateral ribs using fixation plates and subperiosteal wires. The bar applies manual pressure to the anterior chest wall until the desired anatomical configuration is achieved. In their initial series of 40 patients, "highly satisfactory results" were reported with 10/20 patients followed. Complications with this technique reported included pneumothorax requiring chest tube, skin adherence to the bar, seroma formation, wire malfunction, persistent pain, and wound infection. Based on the initial data, the study concluded that the best results could be seen in younger patients whose chest wall was more flexible [32]. It is also important to note that this bar-based technique is not useful in treating chondromanubrial defects where point of maximum protrusion is too superiorly located and there is more limited chest wall compliance.

## Nonoperative Repair

Orthotic bracing was first described in Brazil to treat pectus carinatum in 1992 [33]. Bracing applies continuous direct pressure and counter-pressure over an extended period of time to the deformity enabling long-term remodeling of the costal cartilage. Patients with a compliant chest wall are most responsive to this treatment; thus, the best candidates have been those who are prepubertal between ages 10 and 15 [34]. A variety of bracing devices and protocols have evolved since the initial report in 1992 with complete resolution with the bracing alone to be between 65 and 80 % [15, 35–39].

Regardless of brace type and protocol, the main determinant of success is patient compliance, and thus much of recent research efforts have focused primarily on manufacturing braces that are more comfortable, easily concealed, and with trackable usage [40–43]. Outcomes following orthotic bracing are fairly positive with excellent patient satisfaction and efficacy [44]. Recurrence rates after removal of the brace range between 5 and 15 % [34, 35]. Complications are generally minor and include skin changes, back pain, and hematoma. Of note, case reports of overcorrection to an iatrogenic excavatum have been reported [45]; thus, close follow-up of these patients is required. At many centers, bracing is now considered the first option for intervention offered in patients with chondrogladiolar deformities [46].

## References

1. Shamberger RC, Welch KJ. Surgical correction of pectus carinatum. J Pediatr Surg. 1987;22(1):48–53.
2. Kelly Jr RE, Shamberger RC. Chapter 62—congenital chest wall deformities. In: Coran AG, editor. Pediatric surgery. 7th edn. Philadelphia: Mosby; 2012.p.779–808.http://dx.doi.org/10.1016/B978-0-323-07255-7.00062-3
3. Fonkalsrud EW. Pectus carinatum: the undertreated chest malformation. Asian J Surg. 2003;26(4):189–92. doi:10.1016/S1015-9584(09)60300-6.
4. Lopushinsky SR, Fecteau AH. Pectus deformities: a review of open surgery in the modern era. Semin Pediatr Surg. 2008;17(3):201–8. http://dx.doi.org/10.1053/j.sempedsurg.2008.03.009

5. Desmarais TJ, Keller MS. Pectus carinatum. Curr Opin Pediatr. 2013;25(3):375–81. doi:10.1097/MOP.0b013e3283604088.

6. Papadakis K, Shamberger RC. Congenital chest wall deformities. In: Sellke FW, Del Nido PJ, Swanson SJ, editors. Sabiston & Spencer surgery of the chest. 9th ed. Philadelphia: Elsevier; 2016. p. 399–429.

7. Brodkin HA. Congenital chondrosternal prominence (pigeon breast) a new interpretation. Pediatrics. 1949;3(3):286–95.

8. Robicsek F, Cook JW, Daugherty HK, Selle JG. Pectus carinatum. Coll Works Cardiopulm Dis. 1979;22:65–78.

9. Welch KJ, Vos A. Surgical correction of pectus carinatum (pigeon breast). J Pediatr Surg. 1973;8(5):659–67.

10. Currarino G, Silverman FN. Premature obliteration of the sternal sutures and pigeon-breast deformity. Radiology. 1958;70(4):532–40. doi:10.1148/70.4.532.

11. Ravitch MM. Unusual sternal deformity with cardiac symptoms operative correction. J Thorac Surg. 1952;23(2):138–44.

12. Ravitch MM. Operative correction of pectus carinatum (pigeon breast). Ann Surg. 1960;151(5):705–14.

13. Lester CW. Pigeon breast (pectus carinatum) and other protrusion deformities of the chest of developmental origin. Ann Surg. 1953;137(4):482–9.

14. Robicsek F, Sanger PW, Taylor FH, Thomas MJ. The surgical treatment of chondro-sternal prominence (pectus carinatum). Coll Works Cardiopulm Dis. 1963;66:469–80.

15. Frey AS, Garcia VF, Brown RL, Inge TH, Ryckman FC, Cohen AP, Durrett G, Azizkhan RG. Nonoperative management of pectus carinatum. J Pediatr Surg. 2006;41(1):40–5. http://dx.doi.org/10.1016/j.jpedsurg.2005.10.076

16. Tiller GE, Polumbo PA, Weis MA, Bogaert R, Lachman RS, Cohn DH, Rimoin DL, Eyre DR. Dominant mutations in the type II collagen gene, COL2A1, produce spondyloepimetaphyseal dysplasia, Strudwick type. Nat Genet. 1995;11(1):87–9. doi:10.1038/ng0995-87.

17. Sultan I, Yang S. Congenital chest wall anomalies. Johns Hopkins textbook of cardiothoracic surgery. 2nd ed. New York: McGraw-Hill; 2014.

18. Park CH, Kim TH, Haam SJ, Lee S. Does overgrowth of costal cartilage cause pectus carinatum? A three-dimensional computed tomography evaluation of rib length and costal cartilage length in patients with asymmetric pectus carinatum. Interact Cardiovasc Thorac Surg. 2013;17(5):757–63. doi:10.1093/icvts/ivt321.

19. Steinmann C, Krille S, Mueller A, Weber P, Reingruber B, Martin A. Pectus excavatum and pectus carinatum patients suffer from lower quality of life and impaired body image: a control group comparison of psychological characteristics prior to surgical correction. Eur J Cardiothorac Surg. 2011;40(5):1138–45. doi:10.1016/j.ejcts.2011.02.019.

20. Lees RF, Caldicott JH. Sternal anomalies and congenital heart disease. Am J Roentgenol Radium Ther Nucl Med. 1975;124(3):423–7.

21. Colombani PM. Preoperative assessment of chest wall deformities. Semin Thorac Cardiovasc Surg. 2009;21(1):58–63. doi:10.1053/j.semtcvs.2009.04.003.

22. Robicsek F, Cook JW, Daugherty HK, Selle JG. Pectus carinatum. J Thorac Cardiovasc Surg. 1979;78(1):52–61.

23. Fonkalsrud EW. Surgical correction of pectus carinatum: lessons learned from 260 patients. J Pediatr Surg. 2008;43(7):1235–43. doi:10.1016/j.jpedsurg.2008.02.007.

24. Del Frari B, Schwabegger AH. Ten-year experience with the muscle split technique, bioabsorbable plates, and postoperative bracing for correction of pectus carinatum: the Innsbruck protocol. J Thorac Cardiovasc Surg. 2011;141(6):1403–9. doi:10.1016/j.jtcvs.2011.02.026.

25. Knudsen MV, Grosen K, Pilegaard HK, Laustsen S. Surgical correction of pectus carinatum improves perceived body image, mental health and self-esteem. J Pediatr Surg. 2015;50(9):1472–6. doi:10.1016/j.jpedsurg.2014.11.048.

26. Fonkalsrud EW, Beanes S. Surgical management of pectus carinatum: 30 years' experience. World J Surg. 2001;25(7):898–903.

27. Saxena AK, Willital GH. Surgical repair of pectus carinatum. Int Surg. 1999;84(4):326–30.

28. Colombani PM. Recurrent chest wall anomalies. Semin Pediatr Surg. 2003;12(2):94–9.

29. Kobayashi S, Yoza S, Komuro Y, Sakai Y, Ohmori K. Correction of pectus excavatum and pectus carinatum assisted by the endoscope. Plast Reconstr Surg. 1997;99(4):1037–45.

30. Schaarschmidt K, Kolberg-Schwerdt A, Lempe M, Schlesinger F. New endoscopic minimal access pectus carinatum repair using subpectoral carbon dioxide. Ann Thorac Surg. 2006;81(3):1099–103. doi:10.1016/j.athoracsur.2005.10.042.

31. Kim S, Idowu O. Minimally invasive thoracoscopic repair of unilateral pectus carinatum. J Pediatr Surg. 2009;44(2):471–74. http://dx.doi.org/10.1016/j.jpedsurg.2008.09.020

32. Abramson H, D'Agostino J, Wuscovi S. A 5-year experience with a minimally invasive technique for pectus carinatum repair. J Pediatr Surg. 2009;44(1):118–23. doi:10.1016/j.jpedsurg.2008.10.020. Discussion 123–14.

33. Haje SA, Bowen JR. Preliminary results of orthotic treatment of pectus deformities in children and adolescents. J Pediatr Orthop. 1992;12(6):795–800.

34. Martinez-Ferro M, Fraire C, Bernard S. Dynamic compression system for the correction of pectus carinatum. Semin Pediatr Surg. 2008;17(3):194–200. doi:10.1053/j.sempedsurg.2008.03.008.

35. Lee SY, Lee SJ, Jeon CW, Lee CS, Lee KR. Effect of the compressive brace in pectus carinatum. Eur J Cardiothorac Surg. 2008;34(1):146–9. doi:10.1016/j.ejcts.2008.04.012.

36. Stephenson JT, Du Bois J. Compressive orthotic bracing in the treatment of pectus carinatum: the use of radiographic markers to predict success. J Pediatr

Surg. 2008;43(10):1776–80. doi:10.1016/j.jpedsurg. 2008.03.049.

37. Egan JC, DuBois JJ, Morphy M, Samples TL, Lindell B. Compressive orthotics in the treatment of asymmetric pectus carinatum: a preliminary report with an objective radiographic marker. J Pediatr Surg. 2000;35(8):1183–6.

38. Banever GT, Konefal SH, Gettens K, Moriarty KP. Nonoperative correction of pectus carinatum with orthotic bracing. J Laparoendosc Adv Surg Tech A. 2006;16(2):164–7. doi:10.1089/lap.2006.16.164.

39. Sesia SB, Holland-Cunz S, Hacker FM. Dynamic compression system: an effective nonoperative treatment for pectus carinatum: a single center experience in Basel, Switzerland. Eur J Pediatr Surg. 2016. doi:10.1055/s-0035-1570758.

40. Wong KE, Gorton 3rd GE, Tashjian DB, Tirabassi MV, Moriarty KP. Evaluation of the treatment of pectus carinatum with compressive orthotic bracing using three dimensional body scans. J Pediatr Surg. 2014;49(6):924–7. http://dx.doi.org/10.1016/j.jpedsurg.2014.01.024

41. Kravarusic D, Dicken BJ, Dewar R, Harder J, Poncet P, Schneider M, Sigalet DL. The Calgary protocol for bracing of pectus carinatum: a preliminary report. J Pediatr Surg. 2006;41(5):923–6. doi:10.1016/j.jpedsurg.2006.01.058.

42. Lee RT, Moorman S, Schneider M, Sigalet DL. Bracing is an effective therapy for pectus carinatum: interim results. J Pediatr Surg. 2013;48(1):184–90. doi:10.1016/j.jpedsurg.2012.10.037.

43. Harrison B, Stern L, Chung P, Etemadi M, Kwiat D, Roy S, Harrison MR, Martinez-Ferro M. MyPectus: first-in-human pilot study of remote compliance monitoring of teens using dynamic compression bracing to correct pectus carinatum. J Pediatr Surg. 2015;51(4):608–11. doi:10.1016/j.jpedsurg.2015.11.007.

44. Colozza S, Butter A. Bracing in pediatric patients with pectus carinatum is effective and improves quality of life. J Pediatr Surg. 2013;48(5):1055–9. doi:10.1016/j.jpedsurg.2013.02.028.

45. Haje SA, Haje DP. Overcorrection during treatment of pectus deformities with DCC orthoses: experience in 17 cases. Int Orthop. 2006;30(4):262–7. doi:10.1007/s00264-005-0060-0.

46. APSA Practice Committee. Pectus carinatum guidelines. American Pediatric Surgical Association; 2012

Rajvinder S. Dhamrait and Sundeep S. Tumber

## Key Points

- This chapter will discuss the anesthetic considerations for those patients undergoing repair of chest wall lesions. This will include a description of the preoperative considerations for these patients, intraoperative management, and postoperative issues, including pain control.

## Introduction

The chest wall protects the thoracic and mediastinal organs as well as provides a support structure for the lungs. Lesions of the chest wall are varied, and repair of these lesions can be performed for cosmetic reasons or to prevent the development or worsening of cardiopulmonary symptoms. Some lesions are specific to childhood, while others are also found in adults (Table 5.1) [1].

R.S. Dhamrait, B.M., D.C.H., F.C.A.R.C.S.I., F.R.C.A (✉)
Department of Anesthesiology and Pain Medicine, University of California, Davis School of Medicine, UC Davis Children's Hospital, PSSB Ste 1200, 4150 V Street, Sacramento, CA 95817, USA
e-mail: rsdhamrait@ucdavis.edu

S.S. Tumber, D.O.
Shriners Hospitals for Children—Northern California, 2425 Stockton Boulevard, Sacramento, CA 95817, USA

The pediatric patient will typically undergo physical examination and radiological investigation of the lesion prior to any surgery. Modalities such as ultrasound, computerized tomography (CT), and magnetic resonance imaging (MRI) may be used for confirmation and assessment of the lesion, and the patient may need an anesthetic to facilitate these investigations. The identification of these patients and their subsequent management involves a multidisciplinary approach, with the anesthesiologist, surgeon, intensivist, and allied healthcare professionals (HCP) working closely to ensure a successful outcome.

This chapter will discuss the perioperative anesthetic management of these patients with a focus on analgesic management.

## Management of Anesthesia

### Preanesthetic Assessment

The pediatric patient will need a thorough evaluation prior to induction of anesthesia. The preanesthetic interview allows for a full risk assessment of the patient, investigations, and discussion of the anesthetic plan. Electrocardiography (ECG), echocardiography, and pulmonary function tests should be reviewed where available and relevant. The extent of cardiac and/or pulmonary dysfunction must be determined, and optimization of the patient should occur prior to proceeding to

© Springer International Publishing Switzerland 2017
G.W. Raff, S. Hirose (eds.), *Surgery for Chest Wall Deformities*,
DOI 10.1007/978-3-319-43926-6_5

**Table 5.1** Classification of pediatric chest wall lesions

| |
|---|
| 1. Congenital abnormalities |
| (a) Prominent costal cartilage |
| (b) Pectus excavatum |
| (c) Pectus carinatum |
| 2. Infection |
| (a) Bacterial |
| (b) Fungal |
| 3. Autoimmune |
| (a) Chronic recurrent multifactorial osteomyelitis (CRMO) |
| 4. Neoplasms |
| (a) Soft tissue tumors |
| • Benign |
| – Infantile hemangioma |
| – Infantile fibrous hamartoma |
| – Inflammatory myofibroblastic pseudotumor |
| • Malignant |
| – Rhabdomyosarcoma |
| – Peripheral nerve sheath tumors |
| – Pleuropulmonary blastomas |
| (b) Osseous tumors |
| • Benign |
| – Osteoid osteoma |
| – Osteochondroma |
| – Fibrodysplasia |
| – Mesenchymal hamartoma |
| • Malignant |
| – Ewing sarcoma |
| – Osteosarcoma |
| (c) Metastatic tumors |
| 5. Trauma |
| (a) Accidental |
| (b) Nonaccidental |

Baez JC, Lee EY, Restrepo R et al. (2013) [1]

surgery. The need for blood transfusion should be determined and appropriate samples sent for preparation of blood products. This focused assessment can occur on the day of surgery or in a specialty clinic a few days prior to surgery. Specialty, preanesthetic clinics have shown to reduce hospital costs, reduce cancellations of surgery, and have increased quality of care and rapport with families [2]. Conditions that increase risk to the patient receiving general anesthesia include sleep-disordered breathing, diabetes mellitus, obesity, and recent/concurrent illnesses especially upper respiratory infections (URI) [3].

## Premedication

Preoperative anxiety, seen in at least 60 % of pediatric patients, can lead to a difficult separation from parents, increased stress at induction, worsening postoperative pain, emergence delirium, and psychological and cognitive disturbance for up to 1 week after surgery [4, 5]. Separation anxiety begins around 8 months of age. Use of allied health care professionals including certified child life specialists can limit anxiolysis premedication use, but most children over 8 months old until aged 6 will receive anxiolysis premedication. However, it may be contraindicated in children with severe cardiac, respiratory, or neurological compromise. The common agents can be given by oral (PO), intramuscular (IM), or transmucosal (nasal, buccal) routes, with each route chosen affected by dosing amounts and time given to take effect [6]. If intravenous (i.v.) access is secured preoperatively, the drug can be given by this route.

Benzodiazepines, especially midazolam, cause sedation, amnesia, and anxiolysis, and can be given by PO, intranasal, or IM. It is effective and has a short duration of action, but can have a paradoxical effect in some children [4]. It also has an unpleasant taste and typically reaches a ceiling dose of 20 mg.

Ketamine is another popular agent that can be used as a sole premedicant or can be mixed with another agent, especially midazolam. Mixing the two agents allows for a PO premedicant in the heavier child. Ketamine is an *N-Methyl-*d-*aspartate* (NMDA) receptor antagonist, causing dissociative anesthesia with sedative and analgesic properties. However, it also has side effects, such as increased salivation, hallucinations, and postoperative psychological disturbances [7].

$\alpha$2-Adrenoceptor agonists, such as clonidine and dexmedetomidine, provide all the benefits of premedication without respiratory depression. A 2014 meta-analysis compared dexmedetomidine to other agents. Of 171 studies, 11 allowed comparison of agents and revealed that dexmedetomidine resulted in enhanced preoperative sedation and decreased postoperative pain when compared to midazolam [8].

Premedication may also include inhaled bronchodilators, especially in those patients with a history of reactive airways disease or with concurrent/recent URI [9].

## Monitoring

Applied prior to induction, this should include ECG, pulse oximetry, and noninvasive BP (NIBP) monitoring. More complex monitors can be used as dictated by the associated cardiopulmonary dysfunction. Near-infrared spectroscopy (NIRS) is an absorptive spectrographic method of measuring regional cerebral and somatic oxygenation ($rSO_2$). It measures saturation in both venous and arterial blood and represents an average blood and tissue saturation. $rSO_2$ is affected by changes in oxygen delivery and consumption, and values more than 20 % below baseline or less than an absolute value of 40 % are associated with slowing of EEG potentials and neurological damage. It provides valuable trend monitoring and can be used to assess anesthesia depth [10]. Invasive blood pressure monitoring may be secured as needed.

## Intraoperative Anesthesia Considerations

The choice between a monitored gaseous induction or i.v. induction of anesthesia is patient dependent. In those children without venous access, gaseous induction using sevoflurane, a highly fluorinated methyl isopropyl ether, in an oxygen/air mix of varying ratios is convenient with an early placement of an i.v. cannula once anesthesia is induced. Supplement of the anesthetic with incremental doses of i.v drugs can follow. In other children, an i.v. cannula placed awake may be more desirable. Sevoflurane causes minimal myocardial depression or arrhythmogenesis, but can cause a slight fall in SVR. Heart rate is maintained at standard doses but bradycardia and hypoventilation will occur at higher concentrations.

Nitrous Oxide ($N_2O$) has been in anesthetic use for 150 years, with the benefit of reducing the concentration of inhaled anesthesia needed. It is an antagonist to the NMDA receptor and may reduce postsurgical chronic pain [11]. However, $N_2O$ will expand closed air spaces and so should be avoided where pneumothoraces could occur.

Intravenous anesthesia agents, such as ketamine, etomidate, and propofol, are used to induce anesthesia or supplement a gaseous induction of anesthesia. Each has advantages and disadvantages, but generally i.v. agents have less effect on inhibition on the compensatory hypoxic pulmonary vasoconstriction (HPV) compared to inhaled anesthetics [12]. HPV acts to divert blood from underventilated areas of the lungs, as occur with lung retraction and collapse of the dependent lung in patients in the lateral decubitus position, and diverting this blood to better ventilated areas, thereby reducing V/Q mismatch. Etomidate has hemodynamic stability but is associated with adrenal suppression. Propofol is frequently used in the stable patient but does decrease systemic vascular resistance (SVR) and mean arterial pressure (MAP). Ketamine increases blood pressure, heart rate, and cardiac output by stimulating the release of endogenous catecholamines. It does not affect SVR and does not increase pulmonary vascular resistance (PVR) in children.

Dexmedetomidine is a highly selective α2-adrenoceptor agonist with sedative, anxiolytic, and analgesic properties and minimal effects on respiratory drive. Effects at central α2A and imidazoline-1 receptors result in a reduction in the sympathetic outflow from the locus ceruleus causing decreases in heart rate and SVR, while α2B-adrenoceptors' stimulation in the peripheral vasculature causes an initial increase in SVR. In addition to a decrease in heart rate and SVR, it also shows antiarrhythmic tendencies, slowing conduction through the atrioventricular node and sinoatrial node. Cortisol, epinephrine, norepinephrine, and glucose levels all have been shown to decrease with its use. It has been used successfully in early tracheal extubation following surgery and it may also have a neuronal protective effect [13–15]. Its use also decreases postoperative emergence delirium [16].

Opiates are hemodynamically stable as adjuncts to the induction agent and act to suppress the stress response associated with surgery as well as providing analgesia to the patient. An infusion of remifentanil, an ultrashort acting opioid, is a useful adjunct with a reliable context-sensitive half time of 3–9 min, regardless of duration of infusion.

Airway management for these cases will, in most cases, include muscle relaxation and intubation of the trachea. Nondepolarizing, competitive neuromuscular blockers (NMB) are used for muscle relaxation and act at the acetylcholine (ACh) receptor. The choice between aminosteroid (rocuronium, vecuronium) and benzylisoquinolinium (cisatracurium) may be determined by underlying patient factors or by anesthesiologist. The recent addition of sugammadex, the first selective relaxant binding agent to reverse the effect of aminosteroids, was introduced to the US market in December 2015. Sugammadex, a gamma-cyclodextrin, forms a 1:1 inclusion complex with aminosteroid molecules and has no effect on acetylcholinesterase concentration. It binds to free aminosteroid molecules in the plasma, encourages aminosteroid at the ACh receptor to unbind and move back into the plasma where it is bound as well [17]. Although not recommended for pediatric use by the manufacturer, sugammadex has been successfully studied in this population [18, 19].

Intrathoracic surgical procedures may need lung isolation and one-lung ventilation (OLV). OLV is not typically needed in chest wall surgery, where regular tracheal intubation and bilateral lung ventilation is sufficient. Patient positioning will be determined by the location of the chest wall lesion, and appropriate pressure point padding will be needed.

Pectus deformities are the commonest chest wall deformity seen, with preponderance for males. Pectus excavatum constitutes the majority of these lesions, and repair is by insertion of rigid metal bars in the thoracic cavity, deep to the sternum and costal cartilages (Nuss procedure). This minimally invasive procedure, assisted with use of thoracoscopy, is performed for cosmetic reasons and worsening cardiopulmonary dysfunction, and the repair is performed after puberty, where body image issues and rates of recurrence can be minimized [20]. Intraoperative concerns during the Nuss procedure include dysrhythmias, lung compression, and bleeding [20]. Pain is often worse with the older patient where the repair can be more difficult.

Once chest wall surgery is complete, deep extubation of the trachea will avoid coughing and straining of the patient, reducing the risk of developing subcutaneous emphysema, and an erect chest X-ray should be taken in the recovery room to exclude the presence of pneumothorax or hemothorax [20].

## Pain Management for Chest Wall Surgery

Postoperative pain management of chest wall procedures can be challenging and often requires a multimodal approach. Continuous chest wall movement during respiration and coughing, and nerve and rib disruption from surgical trauma contribute to the severity of the pain. This may adversely affect pulmonary function and cause marked respiratory impairment. Adequate postoperative pain control importantly allows for deep coughing to clear secretions, which prevent atelectasis and pneumonia [21, 22].

This section will discuss the variety of drugs and methods of administration available. The drugs used can be classified into:

1. Opioid analgesia
2. Non-opioid analgesia
3. Analgesic adjuncts
4. Regional analgesia
5. Cryoablation

Nonpharmacological, adjunctive therapies have also been utilized successfully in this patient population to reduce pain scores and should always be considered where appropriate [23, 24]. These include hypnosis and certified child life specialists helping patients cope with postoperative pain issues.

## Opioid Analgesia

Opioid medications are the mainstay for analgesia after most surgical procedures. While very effective, opioids can have multiple adverse side effects. In thoracic surgery, the deleterious side effects of opioid analgesia on pulmonary function are especially significant. Large dose systemic opioids cause sedation and affect the adequacy of respiratory function [23–25]. Patients that receive systemic versus epidural opioids have decreased forced vital capacity and peak expiratory flow rates [26].

Constipation frequently occurs when taking opioid medications and may occur in as many as 40–95 % of people [27]. Nausea and vomiting occurs in 25 % of patients receiving opioids due to the reduced peristaltic activity of the gastrointestinal system [28]. Gastrointestinal bleeding, which is commonly associated with NSAID medications, may also occur from opioids with the rate of bleeding in elderly patients using equaling that of NSAID medications [29]. Additional major side effects of opioids include impaired recovery from surgery, cognitive impairment, urinary retention, pruritus, hypogonadism, hyperalgesia, tolerance, and addiction [30].

Inadequate pain control can lead to poor cough, slower recovery, delayed mobilization, and longer length of hospital stay [22]. Systemic opioid administration as the sole pain modality may not be adequate to treat the intense postoperative pain associated with intrathoracic or chest wall surgery. Thus opioids must often be combined with other non-opioid medications and treatment modalities to minimize side effects while providing adequate analgesia.

## Non-opioid Analgesia

Nonsteroidal anti-inflammatory drugs (NSAIDs) inhibit the enzyme cyclooxygenase (COX), reduce the production of prostaglandins at the site of tissue injury, and decrease inflammation. In addition to their peripheral effect, NSAIDs have a spinal effect by blocking the hyperalgesic response mediated by spinal glutamate and substance P [31]. The analgesic and opioid sparing effects of NSAIDs have been shown to improve the quality of intercostal and epidural analgesia [32–34]. Intravenous ketorolac administered either preemptively before

thoracotomy or postoperatively reduces PCA morphine requirements by 36 % and 17 %, respectively, with no difference in blood loss [35]. In patients managed with a thoracic epidural for the Nuss procedure, ketorolac has been shown to be beneficial for breakthrough pain [34]. NSAIDs are beneficial in alleviating non-incisional pain, such as shoulder and chest tube pain, which is difficult to control with epidural opioid analgesia [36]. NSAIDs can reduce the incidence of opioid-related adverse effects such as respiratory depression, nausea, and vomiting. Side effects of NSAIDS include bronchospasm, acute renal failure, and possibly increased surgical bleeding secondary to altered platelet function.

Acetaminophen exerts its analgesic effects by blocking central prostaglandin synthesis, reducing substance P-induced hyperalgesia, suppressing signal transduction in the spinal cord, and acting on cannabinoid receptors [37, 38]. It can be administered orally, rectally, or intravenously. Postoperative acetaminophen reduces morphine consumption by greater than 30 % after major orthopedic surgery [39]. As with NSAIDs, acetaminophen decreases postthoracotomy shoulder pain when given preemptively and regularly during the first 48 postoperative hours in patients who have received thoracic epidural analgesia [36, 40]. After thoracotomy, use of acetaminophen along with ketorolac and a thoracic epidural reduces the daily dose of epidural medications, improves analgesia, and reduces the incidence of opioid-induced adverse reactions [41]. In an analysis of 21 human studies enrolling over 1900 patients, acetaminophen when combined with NSAIDs, was more effective for treating postoperative pain than either acetaminophen alone or NSAIDs alone [42]. To avoid hepatotoxicity, the maximum daily acetaminophen dose in adults is 4000 mg, and in children 75 mg/kg/day, although doses should be reduced in neonates [43, 44].

## Analgesic Adjuncts

Analgesic adjuncts have been shown to reduce the opioid consumption and reduce the intensity of pain in the perioperative period. Some adjuncts are given by the enteral route only, while others can be given by i.v. infusion and continued into the postoperative period.

## Ketamine

Ketamine, described earlier as a premedicant and an i.v. anesthetic agent, also has analgesic properties in subanesthetic doses. It may prevent the development of opioid-induced hyperalgesia (OIH) and tolerance that can lead to the development of increased postoperative pain and chronic pain states [45]. OIH is a paradoxical response whereby a patient receiving opioids for the treatment of pain can become more sensitive to certain painful stimuli. The type of pain experienced might be the same as the underlying pain or might be different from the original underlying pain [46].

Ketamine for general anesthesia is usually administered intravenously at a dose of 1–2 mg/kg and for procedural sedation at a dose of 0.5 mg/kg IV. Analgesic and antihyperalgesic properties of ketamine are obtained by low-dose infusion at a dose range of 0.15–0.25 mg/kg/h [45]. Low (subanesthetic) doses of ketamine have a small incidence of side effects including dysphoria and hallucinations (1 %), nightmares (2.5 %), visual disturbances (6.2 %), and pleasant dreams (18 %). Side effects can be managed by dose reduction and the use of benzodiazepines [45, 47].

Following the Nuss procedure, a low-dose postoperative ketamine infusion (0.15 mg/kg/h), added to a pain regimen of i.v. hydromorphone PCA and ketorolac, significantly reduced opioid demand and pruritus without an increase in side effects [48]. In a similar trial, a low-dose ketamine infusion added to an i.v. fentanyl PCA resulted in reduced pain scores, consumption of fentanyl, and incidence of nausea and vomiting [49]. The addition of low-dose i.v. ketamine to a regimen of ropivacaine and morphine, by continuous thoracic epidural, has been shown to improve analgesia in postthoracotomy patients [50]. In thoracotomy patients post-lobectomy, desaturation below 90 %, decrease in forced expiratory volume in 1 s, and morphine consumption were lower when a ketamine infusion was added to PCA morphine [51]. In a Cochrane database review of 37 randomized

control trials (2240 participants), perioperative subanesthetic doses of ketamine reduced rescue analgesic requirements, pain intensity, or both. Ketamine reduced 24-h PCA morphine consumption and postoperative nausea and vomiting with adverse effects being mild or absent [52, 53]. Unlike the opioids, low-dose ketamine does not depress respirations. Its benefits, as part of a multimodal pain regimen, include lower opioid demand, decreased pain scores, decreased nausea and vomiting, and decreased pruritus.

## α2-Adrenoceptor Agonists

Dexmedetomidine and clonidine are useful adjuncts in perioperative pain management [54, 55]. Both have been extensively studied in both adult and pediatric populations, although studies in chest wall and intrathoracic surgeries are limited. They both provide sedation and analgesia, with dexmedetomidine having eight times more affinity for the α2-adrenoceptor.

Dexmedetomidine has multiple roles in the perioperative setting. It is used as a premedicant [8], discussed previously, and is very effective in reducing emergence delirium [16]. It has used in sedation for painless procedures, and in painful procedures when used with other medications. As an analgesic, given by i.v. infusion, it has been shown to reduce postoperative opioid requirements, but it is not as effective in reducing pain scores when used as a sole agent [56]. When used as an adjunct with epidural analgesia, it prolongs local anesthesia effect, reduces pain scores, and lowers rescue analgesic requirements [57]. It has been used for opiate withdrawal syndrome. Bradycardia and hypotension can occur, which may limit their use, and sudden cessation can cause rebound hypertension.

## Gabapentinoids

Gabapentin and pregabalin are considered first line therapy for neuropathic pain, but may have a role in acute perioperative pain control. They both work by binding to the $\alpha_2\delta_1$ subunit of presynaptic voltage-dependent calcium channels. These channels are found in the central nervous system and spinal cord dorsal horn, and their activation increases the release of excitatory neurotransmitters. Blockade of these channels therefore reduces this release. Both medications are administered orally with bioavailability inversely proportional to the oral dose. Children under 5 years of age need a 30 % increase in dose to achieve appropriate plasma concentrations [58]. Gabapentin is absorbed in the duodenum, while pregabalin in the majority of the small intestine. Both bypass the liver and are excreted mostly unchanged by the kidneys. Side effects include sedation, dizziness, confusion, and ataxia.

Published results of gabapentin use in adult thoracic surgery have shown that preoperative single-dosing regimes may not be effective in reducing overall opioid use and that continued dosing up to 6 months after surgery may not reduce pain scores and postthoracotomy pain when compared to placebo [59, 60].

In 2010, Rusy et al. studied gabapentin use in pediatric patients undergoing spinal fusion. A single preoperative dose of gabapentin 15 mg/kg was given to the study group and continued for 5 days postoperatively at 5 mg/kg every 8 h. This was compared to placebo, and they found that, on postoperative day 0 and day 1, morphine consumption was lower in the study group, although no difference thereafter. There was no difference in the opioid adverse effects [61]. The importance of postoperative dosing of gabapentin was highlighted in a study of 36 children undergoing spinal surgery in Toronto, where no statistical difference was seen in opioid use when only a single preoperative dose was given [62]. In contrast to this, Amani et al. used a single dose of gabapentin in children undergoing tonsillectomy and found that pain scores were lower in this group when compared to bupivacaine infiltration and i.v. meperidine use [63].

## Magnesium

Magnesium is used in clinical practice to treat electrolyte imbalance, to antagonize calcium, in the treatment of pregnancy-induced hypertension, and in the treatment of refractory bronchospasm. It is also used in the treatment of Torsade de Pointes polymorphic ventricular tachycardia. In increasing dose, magnesium can cause muscle weakness and cardiovascular effects including hypotension, bradycardia, and cardiac arrest.

As an antagonist of the NMDA receptor, it may have some benefit as an opioid-sparing adjunct. In a study of 68 adult patients undergoing elective thoracotomy, an initial dose of 50 mg/kg followed by 500 mg/h intraoperative and for 24 h postoperatively reduced intraoperative analgesia requirements and the postoperative pain scores [64]. It appears not to reduce the risk of supraventricular arrhythmias associated with thoracotomy [65]. In a study of 50 adult patients undergoing gynecological surgery, the use of magnesium reduced the need for intraoperative muscle relaxation, improved postoperative pain scores, and lowered opioid consumption [66].

In pediatric patients, magnesium has been successfully used as an adjunct to epidural analgesia [67] and as an i.v. adjunct to reduce pain scores and opioid use in children with cerebral palsy undergoing orthopedic surgery [68]. However, a prospective study in 2015 found no benefit from the use of magnesium in children undergoing tonsillectomy [69], unlike in adult patients [70]. Although reducing the rate of coughing after tonsillectomy, magnesium does not decrease laryngospasm rates [71].

## Regional Analgesia

### Epidural Analgesia

After a thoracic procedure, there is considerable pain and impairment in pulmonary function. Thoracic epidurals are widely regarded as the "gold standard" for analgesia following thoracic surgery. Epidural analgesia reduces pain and improves pulmonary function by restoring the vital capacity and functional residual capacity to near preoperative levels [26, 72]. Epidural local anesthetics are usually combined with epidural opioids which results in satisfactory pain control, earlier return to ambulation, lower overall opioid requirements, and reduced morbidity when compared to i.v. opioids [25, 26, 72, 73]. Epidural opioids work by binding to opiate receptors in the spinal cord. Morphine, hydromorphone, and fentanyl are the most commonly administered epidural narcotics and are usually administered via continuous infusion. Hydrophilic opioids, such as morphine and hydromorphone, diffuse widely and thus can be administered at either the thoracic or lumbar level to provide pain relief for thoracic procedures [25]. Lipophilic opioids, such as fentanyl, are more effective and smaller doses are required when administered at the thoracic region versus the lumbar region [74]. The most common local anesthetics used in epidural mixtures include bupivacaine and ropivacaine. The efficacy of ropivacaine is similar to that of bupivacaine and it has reduced potential for central nervous system and cardiac toxicity and causes less motor blockade. This may prove to be of benefit for patient mobilization and improvement of respiratory therapy [75, 76].

Risks of epidural placement include infection, nerve damage, drug error, hypotension, and cardiopulmonary arrest [77]. The incidence of respiratory depression after epidural narcotic administration has been reported to be 0.25–0.40 %, and risk factors include age greater than 70 years, presence of pulmonary disease, a thoracic-level epidural, administration of hydrophilic opioids, and concomitant administration of systemic opioids [78]. All patients receiving epidural narcotics should be monitored for respiratory depression for up to 24 h after discontinuation. Other side effects of epidural narcotics include nausea, vomiting, pruritus, and urinary retention. A low-dose naloxone infusion at 1 mcg/kg/h can reduce opioid-related side effects without reversing analgesia [79].

Not all patients will be candidates for epidural catheter placement. Patients who have undergone previous operations on the spine, or are morbidly obese, may not have anatomy suitable for placement of an epidural catheter. Coagulopathy, sepsis, or overlying skin disorders may also be contraindications to its use. Epidural analgesia management also has implications for anesthesia resources, to titrate drug dosing and manage the side effects associated with its use.

## Paravertebral Block

The paravertebral space lies adjacent to the vertebral column and contains thoracic spinal nerves, with their branches, as well as the sympathetic trunk. A paravertebral block (PVB) results in ipsilateral analgesia for unilateral surgeries on the trunk. Bilateral placement can result in effective analgesia of the entire thoracic wall. PVBs can provide equivalent analgesia, a more favorable side effect profile, lessened risk of thoracic neurologic injury, and a lower failure rate when compared to a thoracic epidural [80–84]. Ultrasound guidance can be used to help identify the paravertebral space, needle and catheter placement, and spread of the local anesthetic. The spread of local anesthetic alongside the spine to adjacent paravertebral spaces, anterior to the transverse processes, produces a multilevel block of the chest wall [85]. Bilateral PVB catheters result in equivalent opioid consumption and pain scores when compared to thoracic epidural for postoperative pain management in pediatric patients undergoing Nuss procedures [86]. Complications include technique failure (6.1 %), inadvertent vascular puncture (6.8 %), hypotension (4 %), hematoma (2.4 %), epidural or intrathecal spread (1 %), pleural puncture (0.8 %), and pneumothorax (0.5 %) [87].

## Placement of Subcutaneous Catheters

Analgesia of the thoracic region can be achieved by the intraoperative placement of subcutaneous catheters that deliver local anesthetic just below the incision site or along the intercostal nerves. An *ON-Q* Pain Relief System (I-Flow Corp; Lake Forest, California) can be used for this application. The system consists of an elastomeric pump that holds local anesthetic and is connected by an adjustable flow-limiting valve attached to a soaker hose, to allow for the continuous infusion of local anesthetic to nearby tissues.

The use of the *ON-Q* Pain Relief System as part of a multimodal approach to postoperative pain control has been shown to decrease narcotic use, patient's perception of pain, and length of hospital stay in patients undergoing median sternotomy, thoracotomy, and abdominal surgery [88–91]. Two trials comparing the *ON-Q* Pain Relief System and thoracic epidural for postthoracotomy patients demonstrated similar pain relief and need for on-demand analgesia [92, 93]. A recent retrospective analysis by Choudry et al. compared the use of a continuous chest wall ropivacaine infusion as a part of a multimodal pain regimen to thoracic epidural catheter placement for children undergoing the Nuss procedure. In comparison to the group with the thoracic epidural, the group with continuous subcutaneous catheters had comparable pain control, reduced nausea and vomiting, shorter operating room times, and shorter hospital stay [91]. The advantages of the *ON-Q* system over the placement of a thoracic epidural include ease of placement, less labor intense pain control, and the avoidance of risks associated with a thoracic epidural previously discussed.

## Cryoablation

Pain after chest wall surgery can persist for several months. Cryoanalgesia involves the perioperative freezing of intercostal nerves to reduce thoracic incisional pain. The loss of sensory and motor function that follows cryoanalgesia usually lasts 1–6 months [94]. The intercostal nerve at the incision and two intercostal nerves above and below that are frozen to the −50 to −70 °C range for 90–120 s. Degeneration after freezing and postoperative regeneration of the nerve occurs from the cryoablation site towards the sternum [95, 96]. The risk of pneumothorax using a "blind" approach is as high as 7 % [94]. To reduce the risk of pneumothorax the technique is performed under direct vision, via an open or video-assisted thorascopic approach, or with ultrasound [97–99] (Fig. 5.1). The advantages of a thoracoscopic approach include the use of readily available instruments, direct visualization, and precise placement of the cryoprobe [97] (Fig. 5.2).

Cryoanalgesia was initially proposed as a pain management technique in the mid 1970s but concerns about the risk of development of subsequent chronic neuralgia from permanent intercostal nerve injury and its effectiveness lead to decreased use of the technique [100–103]. Newer techniques and protocols may decrease the risk of nerve injury [103]. Moorjani et al. randomized 200 patients undergoing thoracotomy to cryoanalgesia or parenteral opioids. There was a statistically significant improvement in postoperative pain scores, decreased use of opioid analgesia, and improvement in respiratory function tests for patients in the cryoanalgesia group. In the same study, the

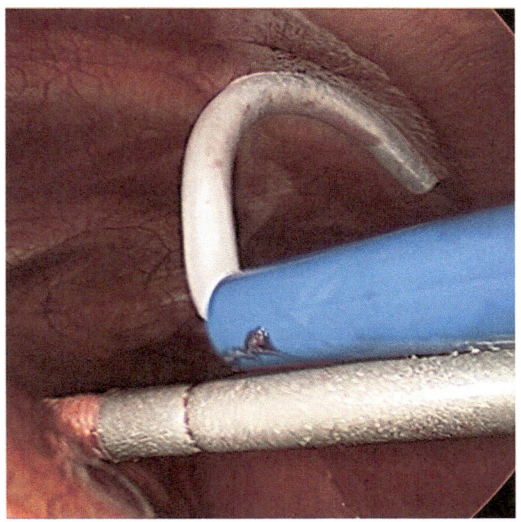

**Fig. 5.1** Cryoanalgesia probe being applied via thoracoscopic approach to chest wall

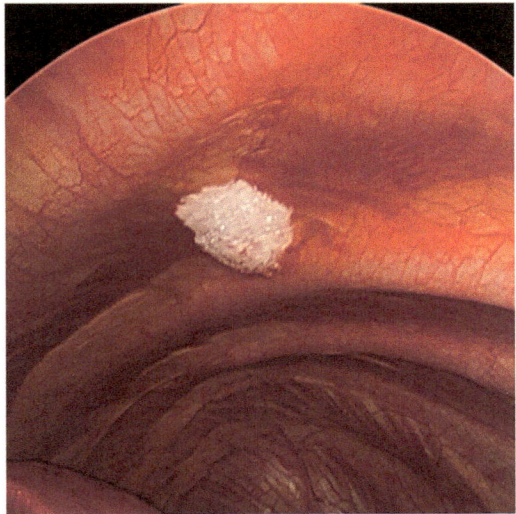

**Fig. 5.2** Resulting freeze area after application of cryoprobe

group anesthetized six dogs and exposed intercostal nerves to a varying duration of cryo-application. The nerves were biopsied and examined histologically at regular intervals over a 6-month period. All nerves had complete recovery and the time taken for recovery was dependant on the period of cryo-application [104]. In another recent study involving 178 lung cancer patients, cryoanalgesia proved to be beneficial in reducing pain, opioid use, and providing long-term postoperative analgesia in patients undergoing lobectomy without any incidence of neuralgia [105]. With the use of newer application devices, techniques, and protocols, cryoanalgesia has been shown to be a safe and effective method for long-term analgesia following thoracic surgery [97, 103–105].

## Summary

- Lesions of the chest wall are varied. Some lesions are specific to childhood, while others are also found in adults. Pectus excavatum constitutes the majority of lesions requiring surgical repair. Repair can be performed for cosmetic reasons or to prevent development or worsening of cardiopulmonary symptoms.
- A focused preoperative assessment should assess cardiopulmonary dysfunction and optimize the patient prior to administration of general anesthesia. Monitoring, both invasive and noninvasive, will be dictated by this preoperative state.
- For pectus excavatum repair, the anesthesiologist should be prepared for risk of dysrhythmia, hemorrhage, and lung compression. Erect chest X-rays should be taken in recovery to exclude postsurgical pneumothorax.
- Analgesia is multimodal. Enteral and parenteral analgesia should be used in conjunction with local anesthetic-based techniques.
- Epidural analgesia remains the "gold standard" of regional analgesia.
- There are an increasing number of studies suggesting that appropriately placed subcutaneous catheters, with infusion of local anesthetic, are as effective as epidural analgesia without the associated risk of epidurals.
- Cryoablation involves the perioperative freezing of intercostal nerves to reduce thoracic incisional pain. There is a risk of development of subsequent chronic neuralgia from permanent intercostal nerve injury, but newer techniques have been shown to be safe and effective method for long-term analgesia following chest wall surgery.

**Acknowledgments** Dr. Dhamrait and Dr. Tumber have no conflict of interest. A check for plagiarism has been performed.

## References

1. Baez JC, Lee EY, Restrepo R, Eisenberg RL. Chest wall lesions in children. AJR Am J Roentgenol. 2013;200(5):W402–19.
2. Gupta A, Gupta N. Setting up and functioning of a pre-anaesthetic clinic. Indian J Anaesth. 2010;54(6):504–7.
3. Tait AR, Malviya S. Anesthesia for the child with an upper respiratory tract infection: still a dilemma? Anesth Analg. 2005;100:59–65.
4. Kain ZN, Wang SM, Mayes LC, Caramico LA, Hofstadter MB. Distress during the induction of anesthesia and postoperative behavioral outcomes. Anesth Analg. 1999;88(5):1042–7.
5. Palermo TM, Drotar D. Prediction of children and postoperative pain: the role of presurgical expectations and anticipatory emotions. J Pediatr Psychol. 1996;21(5):683–98.
6. Strom S. Preoperative evaluation, premedication, and induction of anesthesia in infants and children. Curr Opin Anaesthesiol. 2012;25(3):321–5.
7. Turhanoilu S, Kararmaz A, Ozyilmaz MA, Kaya S, Tok D. Effects of different doses of oral ketamine for premedication of children. Eur J Anaesthesiol. 2003;20:56–60.
8. Peng K, Wu SR, Ji FH, Li J. Premedication with dexmedetomidine in pediatric patients: a systematic review and meta-analysis. Clinics (Sao Paulo). 2014;69(11):777–86.
9. Von Ungern-Sternberg BS, Habre W, Erb TO, Heaney M. Salbutamol premedication in children with a recent respiratory tract infection. Paediatr Anaesth. 2009;19(11):1064–9.
10. Hernandez-Meza G, Izzetoglu M, Osbakken M, Green M, Izzetoglu K. Near-infrared spectroscopy for the evaluation of anesthetic depth. Biomed Res Int. 2015;2015:939418.
11. Chan MT, Wan AC, Gin T, Leslie K, Myles PS. Chronic postsurgical pain after nitrous oxide anesthesia. Pain. 2011;152:2514–20.
12. Lumb AB, Slinger P. Hypoxic pulmonary vasoconstriction: physiology and anesthetic implications. Anesthesiology. 2015;122(4):932–46.
13. Tobias JD, Gupta P, Naguib A, Yates AR. Dexmedetomidine: applications for the pediatric patient with congenital heart disease. Pediatr Cardiol. 2011;32:1075–87.
14. LeRiger M, Naguib A, Gallantowicz M, Tobias JD. Dexmedetomidine controls junctional ectopic

tachycardia during Tetralogy of Fallot repair in an infant. Ann Card Anaesth. 2012;15:224–8.

15. Hammer GB, Drover DR, Cao H, et al. The effects of dexmedetomidine on cardiac electrophysiology in children. Anesth Analg. 2008;106:79–83.

16. Pickard A, Davies P, Birnie K, Beringer R. Systematic review and meta-analysis of the effect of intraoperative α2-adrenergic agonists on postoperative behaviour in children. Br J Anaesth. 2014;112(6):982–90.

17. Srivastava A, Hunter JM. Reversal of neuromuscular block. Br J Anaesth. 2009;103(1):115–29.

18. Bridion® [package insert]. Kenilworth: Merck Pharmaceuticals; 2015.

19. Kara T, Ozbagriacik O, Turk HS, et al. Sugammadex versus neostigmine in pediatric patients: a prospective randomized study. Braz J Anesthesiol. 2014;64(6):400–5.

20. Mavi J, Moore DL. Anesthesia and analgesia for pectus excavatum surgery. Anesthesiol Clin. 2014;32(1):175–84.

21. Sabanathan S, Eng J, Mearns AJ. Alterations in respiratory mechanics following thoracotomy. J R Coll Surg Edinb. 1990;35(3):144–50.

22. Richardson J, Sabanathan S, Shah R. Postthoracotomy spirometric lung function: the effect of analgesia. A review. J Cardiovasc Surg (Torino). 1999;40(3):445–56.

23. Lobe TE. Perioperative hypnosis reduces hospitalization in patients undergoing the Nuss procedure for pectus excavatum. J Laparoendosc Adv Surg Tech. 2007;16(6):639–42.

24. Manworren R, Girard E, Verissimo AM, et al. Hypnosis for postoperative pain management of thoracoscopic approach to repair pectus excavatum: retrospective analysis. J Pediatr Surg Nurs. 2015;4(2):60–9.

25. Cook TM, Riley RH. Analgesia following thoracotomy: a survey of Australian practice. Anaesth Intensive Care. 1997;25(5):520–4.

26. Stone JG, Cozine KA, Wald A. Nocturnal oxygenation during patient-controlled analgesia. Anesth Analg. 1999;89(1):104–10.

27. Soto RG, Fu ES. Acute pain management for patients undergoing thoracotomy. Ann Thorac Surg. 2003;75(4):1349–57.

28. Shulman M, Sandler AN, Bradley JW, Young PS, Brebner J. Postthoracotomy pain and pulmonary function following epidural and systemic morphine. Anesthesiology. 1984;61(5):569–75.

29. Benyamin R, Trescot AM, Datta S, et al. Opioid complications and side effects. Pain Physician. 2008;11(2 Suppl):S105–20.

30. Swegle JM, Logemann C. Management of common opioid-induced adverse effects. Am Fam Physician. 2006;74(8):1347–54.

31. Solomon DH, Rassen JA, Glynn RJ, Lee J, Levin R, Schneeweiss S. The comparative safety of analgesics in older adults with arthritis. Arch Intern Med. 2010;170(22):1968–76.

32. Teater D. The psychological and physical side effects of pain medications. National Safety Council; 2015.

33. Malmberg AB, Yaksh TL. Hyperalgesia mediated by spinal glutamate or substance P receptor blocked by spinal cyclooxygenase inhibition. Science. 1992; 257(5074):1276–9.

34. Singh H, Bossard RF, White PF, Yeatts RW. Effects of ketorolac versus bupivacaine coadministration during patient-controlled hydromorphone epidural analgesia after thoracotomy procedures. Anesth Analg. 1997;84(3):564–9.

35. Carretta A, Zannini P, Chiesa G, Altese R, Melloni G, Grossi A. Efficacy of ketorolac tromethamine and extrapleural intercostal nerve block on postthoracotomy pain. A prospective, randomized study. Int Surg. 1996;81(3):224–8.

36. Densmore JC, Peterson DB, Stahovic LL, et al. Initial surgical and pain management outcomes after Nuss procedure. J Pediatr Surg. 2010;45(9):1767–71.

37. Boussofara M, Mtaallah MH, Bracco D, Sellam MR, Raucoles M. Co-analgesic effect of ketorolac after thoracic surgery. Tunis Med. 2006;84(7):427–31.

38. Burgess FW, Anderson DM, Colonna D, Sborov MJ, Cavanaugh DG. Ipsilateral shoulder pain following thoracic surgery. Anesthesiology. 1993;78(2):365–8.

39. Malviya S, Polaner DM, Berde C. Acute pain. In: Cote CJ, Lerman J, Todres ID, editors. A practice of anesthesia for infants and children. Philadelphia: Saunders Elsevier; 2009. p. 939–78.

40. Andersson DA, Gentry C, Alenmyr L, et al. TRPA1 mediates spinal antinociception induced by acetaminophen and the cannabinoid Δ(9)-tetrahydrocannabiorcol. Nat Commun. 2011;2:551.

41. Sinatra RS, Jahr JS, Reynolds LW, Viscusi ER, Groudine SB, Payen-champenois C. Efficacy and safety of single and repeated administration of 1 gram intravenous acetaminophen injection (paracetamol) for pain management after major orthopedic surgery. Anesthesiology. 2005;102(4):822–31.

42. Mac TB, Girard F, Chouinard P, et al. Acetaminophen decreases early post-thoracotomy ipsilateral shoulder pain in patients with thoracic epidural analgesia: a double-blind placebo-controlled study. J Cardiothorac Vasc Anesth. 2005;19(4):475–8.

43. Uvarov DN, Orlov MM, Levin AV, Sokolov AV, Nedashkovskiĭ EV. [Role of paracetamol in a balanced postoperative analgesia scheme after thoracotomy]. Anesteziol Reanimatol. 2008;(4):46–9.

44. Ong CK, Seymour RA, Lirk P, Merry AF. Combining paracetamol (acetaminophen) with nonsteroidal antiinflammatory drugs: a qualitative systematic review of analgesic efficacy for acute postoperative pain. Anesth Analg. 2010;110(4):1170–9.

45. Shiffman S, Rohay JM, Battista D, et al. Patterns of acetaminophen medication use associated with exceeding the recommended maximum daily dose. Pharmacoepidemiol Drug Saf. 2015;24(9):915–21.

46. Walker SM. Neonatal pain. Paediatr Anaesth. 2014;24(1):39–48.

47. Rakic AM, Golembiewski J. Low-dose ketamine infusion for postoperative pain management. J Perianesth Nurs. 2009;24(4):254–7.

48. Lee M, Silverman SM, Hansen H, Patel VB, Manchikanti L. A comprehensive review of opioid-induced hyperalgesia. Pain Physician. 2011; 14(2):145–61.

49. Elia N, Tramèr MR. Ketamine and postoperative pain—a quantitative systematic review of randomised trials. Pain. 2005;113(1-2):61–70.

50. Min TJ, Kim WY, Jeong WJ, et al. Effect of ketamine on intravenous patient-controlled analgesia using hydromorphone and ketorolac after the Nuss surgery in pediatric patients. Korean J Anesthesiol. 2012;62(2):142–7.

51. Cha MH, Eom JH, Lee YS, et al. Beneficial effects of adding ketamine to intravenous patient-controlled analgesia with fentanyl after the Nuss procedure in pediatric patients. Yonsei Med J. 2012;53(2):427–32.

52. Suzuki M, Haraguti S, Sugimoto K, Kikutani T, Shimada Y, Sakamoto A. Low-dose intravenous ketamine potentiates epidural analgesia after thoracotomy. Anesthesiology. 2006;105(1):111–9.

53. Michelet P, Guervilly C, Hélaine A, et al. Adding ketamine to morphine for patient-controlled analgesia after thoracic surgery: influence on morphine consumption, respiratory function, and nocturnal desaturation. Br J Anaesth. 2007;99(3):396–403.

54. Bell RF, Dahl JB, Moore RA, Kalso E. Perioperative ketamine for acute postoperative pain. Cochrane Database Syst Rev. 2006;1:CD004603.

55. Su F, Hammer GB. Dexmedetomidine: pediatric pharmacology, clinical uses and safety. Expert Opin Drug Saf. 2011;10(1):55–66.

56. Yuen VM. Dexmedetomidine: perioperative applications in children. Paediatr Anaesth. 2010;20(3): 256–64.

57. Schnabel A, Meyer-Frießem CH, Reichl SU, Zahn PK, Pogatzki-Zahn EM. Is intraoperative dexmedetomidine a new option for postoperative pain treatment? A meta-analysis of randomized controlled trials. Pain. 2013;154(7):1140–9.

58. Kaur S, Attri JP, Kaur G, Singh TP. Comparative evaluation of ropivacaine versus dexmedetomidine and ropivacaine in epidural anesthesia in lower limb orthopedic surgeries. Saudi J Anaesth. 2014;8(4):463–9.

59. Haig GM, Bockbrader HN, Wesche DL, et al. Single-dose gabapentin pharmacokinetics and safety in healthy infants and children. J Clin Pharmacol. 2001;41:507–14.

60. Grosen K, Drewes AM, Højsgaard A, Pfeiffer-jensen M, Hjortdal VE, Pilegaard HK. Perioperative gabapentin for the prevention of persistent pain after thoracotomy: a randomized controlled trial. Eur J Cardiothorac Surg. 2014;46(1):76–85.

61. Zakkar M, Frazer S, Hunt I. Is there a role for gabapentin in preventing or treating pain following thoracic surgery? Interact Cardiovasc Thorac Surg. 2013;17(4):716–9.

62. Rusy LM, Hainsworth KR, Nelson TJ, et al. Gabapentin use in pediatric spinal fusion patients: a randomized, double-blind, controlled trial. Anesth Analg. 2010;110(5):1393–8.

63. Mayell A, Srinivasan I, Campbell F, et al. Analgesic effects of gabapentin after scoliosis surgery in children: a randomized controlled trial. Paediatr Anaesth. 2014;24:1239–44.

64. Amani S, Abedinzadeh MR. Effects of oral gabapentin, local bupivacaine and intravenous pethidine on post tonsillectomy pain. Iran J Otorhinolaryngol. 2015;27:343–8.

65. Kogler J. The analgesic effect of magnesium sulfate in patients undergoing thoracotomy. Acta Clin Croat. 2009;48(1):19–26.

66. Saran T, Perkins GD, Javed MA, et al. Does the prophylactic administration of magnesium sulphate to patients undergoing thoracotomy prevent postoperative supraventricular arrhythmias? A randomized controlled trial. Br J Anaesth. 2011; 106(6):785–91.

67. Ryu JH, Kang MH, Park KS, Do SH. Effects of magnesium sulphate on intraoperative anaesthetic requirements and postoperative analgesia in gynaecology patients receiving total intravenous anaesthesia. Br J Anaesth. 2008;100(3):397–403.

68. Kim EM, Kim MS, Han SJ, et al. Magnesium as an adjuvant for caudal analgesia in children. Paediatr Anaesth. 2014;24(12):1231–8.

69. Na HS, Lee JH, Hwang JY, et al. Effects of magnesium sulphate on intraoperative neuromuscular blocking agent requirements and postoperative analgesia in children with cerebral palsy. Br J Anaesth. 2010;104(3):344–50.

70. Benzon HA, Shah RD, Hansen J, et al. The effect of systemic magnesium on postsurgical pain in children undergoing tonsillectomies: a double-blinded, randomized, Placebo-Controlled Trial. Anesth Analg. 2015;121(6):1627–31.

71. Tugrul S, Degirmenci N, Eren SB, Dogan R, Veyseller B, Ozturan O. Analgesic effect of magnesium in post-tonsillectomy patients: a prospective randomised clinical trial. Eur Arch Otorhinolaryngol. 2015;272(9):2483–7.

72. Marzban S, Haddadi S, Naghipour MR, Sayah Varg Z, Naderi Nabi B. The effect of intravenous magnesium sulfate on laryngospasm after elective adenotonsillectomy surgery in children. Anesth Pain Med. 2014;4(1):e15960.

73. Hasenbos MA, Eckhaus MN, Slappendel R, Gielen MJ. Continuous high thoracic epidural administration of bupivacaine with sufentanil or nicomorphine for postoperative pain relief after thoracic surgery. Reg Anesth. 1989;14(5):212–8.

74. Rawal N, Sjöstrand U, Christoffersson E, Dahlström B, Arvill A, Rydman H. Comparison of intramuscular and epidural morphine for postoperative analgesia in the grossly obese: influence on postoperative ambulation and pulmonary function. Anesth Analg. 1984;63(6):583–92.

75. Swaroop NS, Batra YK, Bhardwaj N, Chari P, Ram P. A comparative evaluation of thoracic and lumbar epidural fentanyl for post thoracotomy pain. Ann Card Anaesth. 2002;5(1):53–8.

76. Macias A, Monedero P, Adame M, Torre W, Fidalgo I, Hidalgo F. A randomized, double-blinded comparison of thoracic epidural ropivacaine, ropivacaine/fentanyl, or bupivacaine/fentanyl for postthoracotomy analgesia. Anesth Analg. 2002;95(5):1344–50.

77. Hodgson PS, Liu SS. A comparison of ropivacaine with fentanyl to bupivacaine with fentanyl for postoperative patient-controlled epidural analgesia. Anesth Analg. 2001;92(4):1024–8.

78. Llewellyn N, Moriarty A. The national pediatric epidural audit. Paediatr Anaesth. 2007;17(6):520–33.

79. Gustafsson LL, Schildt B, Jacobsen K. Adverse effects of extradural and intrathecal opiates: report of a nationwide survey in Sweden. 1982. Br J Anaesth. 1998;81(1):86–93.

80. Monitto CL, Kost-byerly S, White E, et al. The optimal dose of prophylactic intravenous naloxone in ameliorating opioid-induced side effects in children receiving intravenous patient-controlled analgesia morphine for moderate to severe pain: a dose finding study. Anesth Analg. 2011;113(4):834–42.

81. Richardson J, Lönnqvist PA, Naja Z. Bilateral thoracic paravertebral block: potential and practice. Br J Anaesth. 2011;106(2):164–71.

82. Scarci M, Joshi A, Attia R. In patients undergoing thoracic surgery is paravertebral block as effective as epidural analgesia for pain management? Interact Cardiovasc Thorac Surg. 2010;10(1):92–6.

83. Kelly RE, Goretsky MJ, Obermeyer R, et al. Twenty-one years of experience with minimally invasive repair of pectus excavatum by the Nuss procedure in 1215 patients. Ann Surg. 2010;252(6):1072–81.

84. Meyer MJ, Krane EJ, Goldschneider KR, Klein NJ. Case report: neurological complications associated with epidural analgesia in children: a report of 4 cases of ambiguous etiologies. Anesth Analg. 2012;115(6):1365–70.

85. Ding X, Jin S, Niu X, Ren H, Fu S, Li Q. A comparison of the analgesia efficacy and side effects of paravertebral compared with epidural blockade for thoracotomy: an updated meta-analysis. PLoS One. 2014;9(5):e96233.

86. Richardson J, Lönnqvist PA. Thoracic paravertebral block. Br J Anaesth. 1998;81(2):230–8.

87. Hall Burton DM, Boretsky KR. A comparison of paravertebral nerve block catheters and thoracic epidural catheters for postoperative analgesia following the Nuss procedure for pectus excavatum repair. Paediatr Anaesth. 2014;24(5):516–20.

88. Naja Z, Lönnqvist PA. Somatic paravertebral nerve blockade. Incidence of failed block and complications. Anaesthesia. 2001;56(12):1184–8.

89. Wheatley GH, Rosenbaum DH, Paul MC, et al. Improved pain management outcomes with continuous infusion of a local anesthetic after thoracotomy. J Thorac Cardiovasc Surg. 2005;130(2):464–8.

90. Barron DJ, Tolan MJ, Lea RE. A randomized controlled trial of continuous extra-pleural analgesia post-thoracotomy: efficacy and choice of local anaesthetic. Eur J Anaesthesiol. 1999;16(4):236–45.

91. Gebhardt R, Mehran RJ, Soliz J, Cata JP, Smallwood AK, Feeley TW. Epidural versus ON-Q local anesthetic-infiltrating catheter for post-thoracotomy pain control. J Cardiothorac Vasc Anesth. 2013;27(3):423–6.

92. Givens VA, Lipscomb GH, Meyer NL. A randomized trial of postoperative wound irrigation with local anesthetic for pain after cesarean delivery. Am J Obstet Gynecol. 2002;186(6):1188–91.

93. Ried M, Schilling C, Potzger T, et al. Prospective, comparative study of the On-Q® PainBuster® postoperative pain relief system and thoracic epidural analgesia after thoracic surgery. J Cardiothorac Vasc Anesth. 2014;28(4):985–90.

94. Choudhry DK, Brenn BR, Sacks K, Reichard K. Continuous chest wall ropivacaine infusion for analgesia in children undergoing Nuss procedure: a comparison with thoracic epidural. Paediatr Anaesth. 2016;26(6):582–9.

95. Green CR, De Rosayro AM, Tait AR. The role of cryoanalgesia for chronic thoracic pain: results of a long-term follow up. J Natl Med Assoc. 2002; 94(8):716–20.

96. CryoA procedure brochure. Cincinnati: AtriCure. http://www.atricure.com

97. Moorjani N, Zhao F, Tian Y, Liang C, Kaluba J, Maiwand MO. Effects of cryoanalgesia on post-thoracotomy pain and on the structure of intercostal nerves: a human prospective randomized trial and a histological study. Eur J Cardiothorac Surg. 2001; 20(3):502–7.

98. Momenzadeh S, Elyasi H, Valaie N, et al. Effect of cryoanalgesia on post-thoracotomy pain. Acta Med Iran. 2011;49(4):241–5.

99. Hunt I, Eaton D, Maiwand O, Anikin V. Video-assisted intercostal nerve cryoablation in managing intractable chest wall pain. J Thorac Cardiovasc Surg. 2010;139(3):774–5.

100. Byas-Smith MG, Gulati A. Ultrasound-guided intercostal nerve cryoablation. Anesth Analg. 2006; 103(4):1033–5.

101. Maiwand O, Makey AR. Cryoanalgesia for relief of pain after thoracotomy. Br Med J (Clin Res Ed). 1981;282(6278):1749–50.

102. Maiwand MO, Makey AR, Rees A. Cryoanalgesia after thoracotomy. Improvement of technique and review of 600 cases. J Thorac Cardiovasc Surg. 1986;92(2):291–5.

103. Roxburgh JC, Markland CG, Ross BA, Kerr WF. Role of cryoanalgesia in the control of pain after thoracotomy. Thorax. 1987;42(4):292–5.

104. Sepsas E, Misthos P, Anagnostopulu M, Toparlaki O, Voyagis G, Kakaris S. The role of intercostal cryoanalgesia in post-thoracotomy analgesia. Interact Cardiovasc Thorac Surg. 2013;16(6): 814–8.

105. Ba YF, Li XD, Zhang X, et al. Comparison of the analgesic effects of cryoanalgesia vs. parecoxib for lung cancer patients after lobectomy. Surg Today. 2014;45(10):1250–4.

# Poland's Syndrome

## Alessandro G. Cusano and Michael S. Wong

## Introduction

Poland's Syndrome, in the classic sense, is the unilateral absence of the sternocostal head of the pectoralis major muscle, ipsilateral breast hypoplasia, and a concomitant, ipsilateral hand deformity. The syndrome has since evolved to encompass a myriad of anomalies, rarely presenting collectively in the same individual. Consistent in all cases, the congenital absence of the sternocostal head of the pectoralis major muscle is pathognomonic for the disease. With few exceptions, Poland's Syndrome represents primarily an aesthetic deformity. Aside from the rare case of cardiopulmonary compromise, surgical intervention is typically delayed until growth is complete. A single-stage approach is preferred, with interdisciplinary collaboration recommended to optimize reconstructive outcomes.

## History

In 1841, 19-year-old Alfred Poland provided a detailed account of an unusual anatomic dissection that he performed as a medical student and anatomy apprentice at Guy's Hospital in London, England. The body was that of 27-year-old convict, George Pelt, who reportedly had difficultly adducting his left arm. Poland's findings would not only provide an explanation for the condition, but inspire a sketch of the cadaver's thorax and a preservation of the subject's hand in the medical museum of Guys Hospital (Fig. 6.1) [1, 2]. Poland's work was later printed in the *Guy's Hospitals Reports* under the title "Deficiency of the pectoral muscles;" [3] and the collection of findings he so astutely described would later serve as the classic description of the syndrome that today bears his name.

It should be noted, however, several reports of similar deformities preceded Poland's [4–6]. No syndrome or eponym existed at the time; and preceding accounts failed to acknowledge the concomitant hand abnormality. It wasn't until 1962, over one hundred years later, that Poland's name was first ascribed to the condition. Patrick Clarkson, a Plastic and Hand Surgeon at Guy's Hospital, coined the term "Poland's Syndactyly" to refer to the simultaneous occurrence of breast hypoplasia and syndactyly that he noted in three of his patients [7, 8]. Five years later, Baudinne

A.G. Cusano, M.D. (✉) • M.S. Wong, M.D.(✉)
Department of Surgery, Division of Plastic Surgery,
University of California, Davis Medical Center,
2221 Stockton Boulevard, Suite 2123, Sacramento,
CA 95817, USA
e-mail: mswong@ucdavis.edu

© Springer International Publishing Switzerland 2017
G.W. Raff, S. Hirose (eds.), *Surgery for Chest Wall Deformities*,
DOI 10.1007/978-3-319-43926-6_6

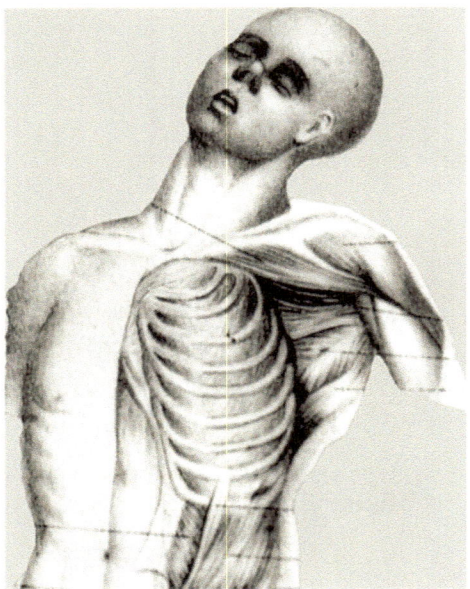
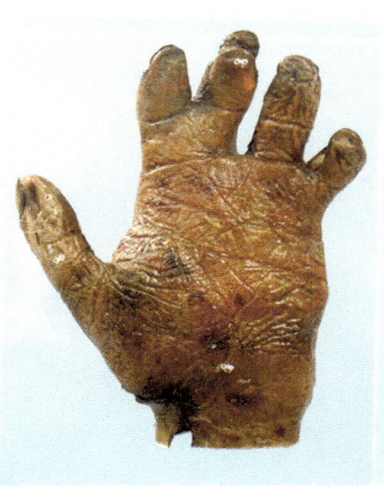

**Fig. 6.1** (*Left*) Illustration made during the 1841 dissection by Alfred Poland and drawn by Poland's friend, Mr. Tilston. [From Poland, A. Deficiency of the pectoral muscles. GuysHospRep.1841;6:191. Note: Guy's Hospital Reports went out of print in 1974 [7].] (*Right*) The left hand of Poland's 1841 subject as it appears today at the Gordon Museum of Guy's Hospital, London. The photo-graph was kindly taken for inclusion [in the article from which this figure was referenced] by William G. J. Edwards, Keeper of the Gordon Museum, Kings College, London, after a recent visit to the museum (and the specimen) by the senior author (A.E.S.) [of the article referenced]. (Used with permission from [2]

and colleagues, in their 1967 publication, referred to the complex as "Poland's Syndrome," an eponym that continues to this day [9].

## Epidemiology

The true incidence of Poland's Syndrome is difficult to estimate due to the variability with which it presents and the differences that occur in the specific patient cohorts. Most studies indicate an average incidence of 1 in 20,000 to 1 in 30,000 live births, with ranges of 1 in 7000 to 1 in 100,000 reported. It is a condition that lends itself to under-reporting, being a predominantly aesthetic deformity and one that is rather easily concealed. Mammography, providing perhaps a more objective measure, has demonstrated an incidence of 1 in 19,000 [10].

Poland's Syndrome is most commonly a right-sided, sporadic, congenital deformity. Familial

cases have been described, but the incidence of such cases is less than 1 %. Single accounts of bilateral muscle agenesis do exist, and the occasional study demonstrating a left-sided predominance has been reported [11]. Males are affected more frequently than females with a ratio of 2:1 to 3:1. Males show a marked predilection for right-sided involvement; females, in contrast, show much less sidedness. In sporadic cases, the pattern of male and right-sided predominance holds true. In familial cases, however, the incidence in males and females is similar; and the deformity presents equally as common on either side in both genders [10, 11].

## Pathogenesis

Although familial cases have been described, Poland's Syndrome is thought to result from events in utero rather than defined inheritance. Its predominantly unilateral, sporadic occurrence lends support to the idea of an intrauterine insult as the inciting factor. This view is further substantiated by a report of Poland's Syndrome in only one sibling of a pair of monozygotic twins [10]. The prevailing etiological theory for Poland's Syndrome favors a vascular origin for the causal intrauterine event.

Bavnick and Weaver suggested the term "subclavian artery supply disruption sequence (SASDS)" to explain the pathogenesis of a group of syndromes that includes Poland's Syndrome. They proposed these conditions resulted from an interruption of early embryonic blood supply in the subclavian or vertebral arteries, or their branches, occurring at or around the sixth week of embryologic development. They further hypothesized that occlusion at specific locations within these vessels produced predictable patterns of defects [12].

With respect to Poland's Syndrome specifically, an early low-flow state to the developing limb bud at the sixth to seventh week of gestation has been suggested with findings of regional vascular hypoplasia corroborating this theory. Decreases in diameter of greater than 50% and reductions in flow velocity have been demonstrated in the subclavian arteries of patients with Poland's Syndrome [12–14]. In their case report of an aborted ipsilateral latissimus dorsi flap in a 17-year-old girl with Poland's Syndrome, Beer et al. present angiographic data demonstrating a hypoplastic, ipsilateral subclavian artery with complete absence of both the ipsilateral thoracoacromial and thoracodorsal branches [15]. Interestingly, the finding of vascular hypoplasia was noted by Alfred Poland, himself. In his initial description, he remarked upon the presence yet diminished size of the thoracic vessels supplying the intercostal spaces [3].

Despite the support for a vascular theory of pathogenesis, skeptics note the sparing of musculoskeletal units on the affected side downstream from the alleged occlusive event as evidence to the contrary of a vascular etiology. An alternative hypothesis is the disruption of the lateral plate mesoderm, from which the pectoralis major muscle develops between 16 and 28 days after fertilization. This disruption has been suggested to account for all defects [10].

The phenotypic mosaicism observed with Poland's Syndrome has been explained in terms of timing of cell death. A lethal mutation of an upper limb bud cell line has been postulated as the inciting event. Early mutation explains the more severe chest wall and limb defects, whereas, later mutations may produce more localized skin and soft tissue anomalies [11].

Finally, reports of familial cases should not be entirely dismissed. Soltan and Holmes suggested a familial clustering of a common factor (e.g. a vascular abnormality) to describe the occurrence of Poland's Syndrome in different members of the two sets of siblings who were first cousins [16]. Sujansky et al. proposed a delayed mutation of an autosomal dominant gene to explain the occurrence in two family members related through three unaffected individuals [17]. The delayed mutation theory does appear consistent with these and other reports of familial cases, accurately accounting for both the vertical transmission from parent to child and for cases of affected siblings with unaffected parents.

## Clinical Features and Classification

The constellation of clinical features that make up Poland's Syndrome is quite variable in its presentation. The sine qua non, however, is the congenital absence of the sternocostal head of the pectoralis major muscle. This feature can present alone, or with ipsilateral chest wall and upper extremity deformities. The extent and involvement of each of these components is variable, such that the syndrome is best regarded as a spectrum that varies with the involvement and severity of the constituent anomalies.

A number of classification systems have been described. Seyfer et al. classify the 63 patients in their series as having either "simple" or "complex" Poland's Syndrome; the "simple" form representing the unilateral absence of the sternocostal head of the pectoralis major muscle, and the "complex" form presenting with the addition of rib and sternal aberrations, muscular displacements, and brachysyndactyly (Figs. 6.2 and 6.3) [2].

Fokin and colleagues divide the syndrome into three groups: "mild (or partial)," "moder-

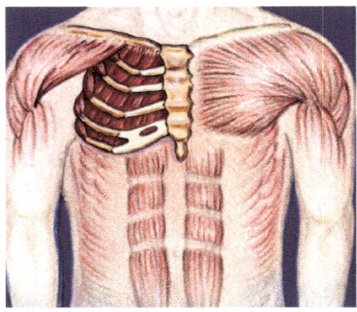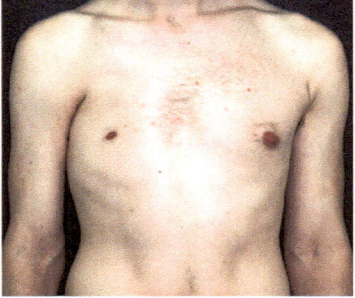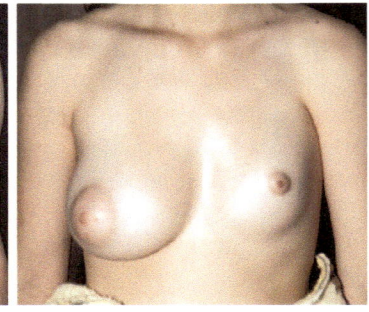

**Fig. 6.2** Simple form of Poland syndrome. (*Left*) Illustration of absence of the right sternocostal head of the pectoralis major muscle. (*Center*) Male patient with right-sided Poland syndrome. (*Right*) Female patient with left-sided Poland syndrome. Note the asymmetric anterior axillary folds. Both sexes usually express concern about the folds and their chest wall asymmetry. (Used with permission from Seyfer, AE.; Fox, JP.; Hamilton, CG. Poland Syndrome: Evaluation and Treatment of the Chest Wall in 63 Patients. Plast Reconstr Surg. 2010; 126(3):902–911)

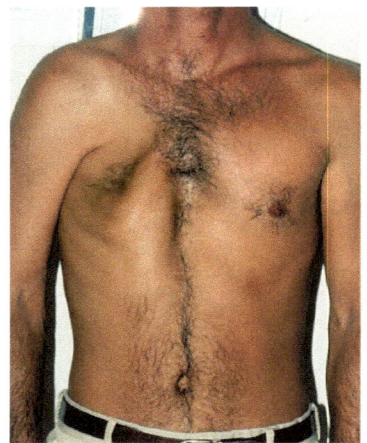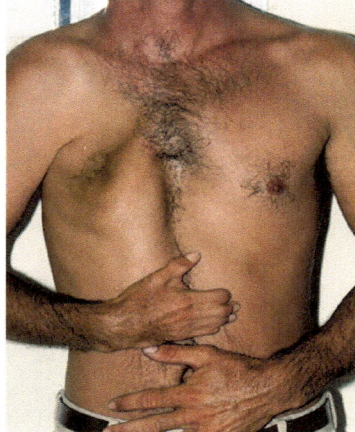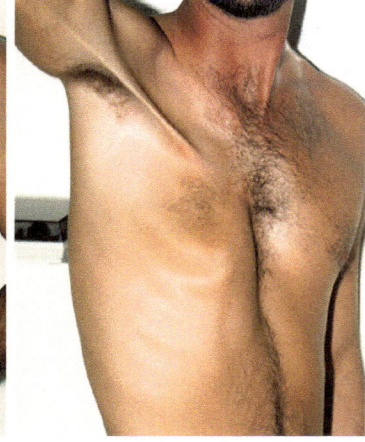

**Fig. 6.3** Complex form of Poland syndrome in a male patient. (*Left*) The right hemithorax is smaller and the cartilaginous portions of the upper ribs are absent. With the arms at the side, the axillary fold deficiency is apparent. (*Center*) The upper extremity components are short and there is a brachysyndactyly (shortened,webbed digits) as described by Poland. (From Seyfer AE, Icochea R, Graeber GM. Poland's anomaly: Natural history and long-term results of chest wall reconstruction in 33 patients. Ann Surg. 1988;208:776–782. Used with permission). (*Right*) An axillary web is present, which may represent a forme fruste of the pectoralis major muscle. This webbing, which can also be observed in the simple form, is sometimes contractile. (Used with permission from Seyfer, AE.; Fox, JP.; Hamilton, CG. Poland Syndrome: Evaluation and Treatment of the Chest Wall in 63 Patients. Plast Reconstr Surg. 2010; 126(3):902–911)

ate (or classic)," and "severe." The "mild (or partial)" form is the equivalent of Seyfer's "simple" designation, representing the sine qua non of the disease. Fokin's "moderate (or classic)" form and Seyfer's "complex" form are also similar in that they represent the features originally noted by Poland in his initial report (i.e. pectoralis muscle aplasia, costochondral hypoplasia, and unilateral brachysyndactyly). Fokin adds an additional group of increased severity which he terms the "severe" form; to distinguish those cases that present with the added complexity of lung herniation, latissismus dorsi and deltoid muscle involvement, dextrocardia, ectrodactyly, and/or renal agenesis (Figs. 6.4 and 6.5) [18].

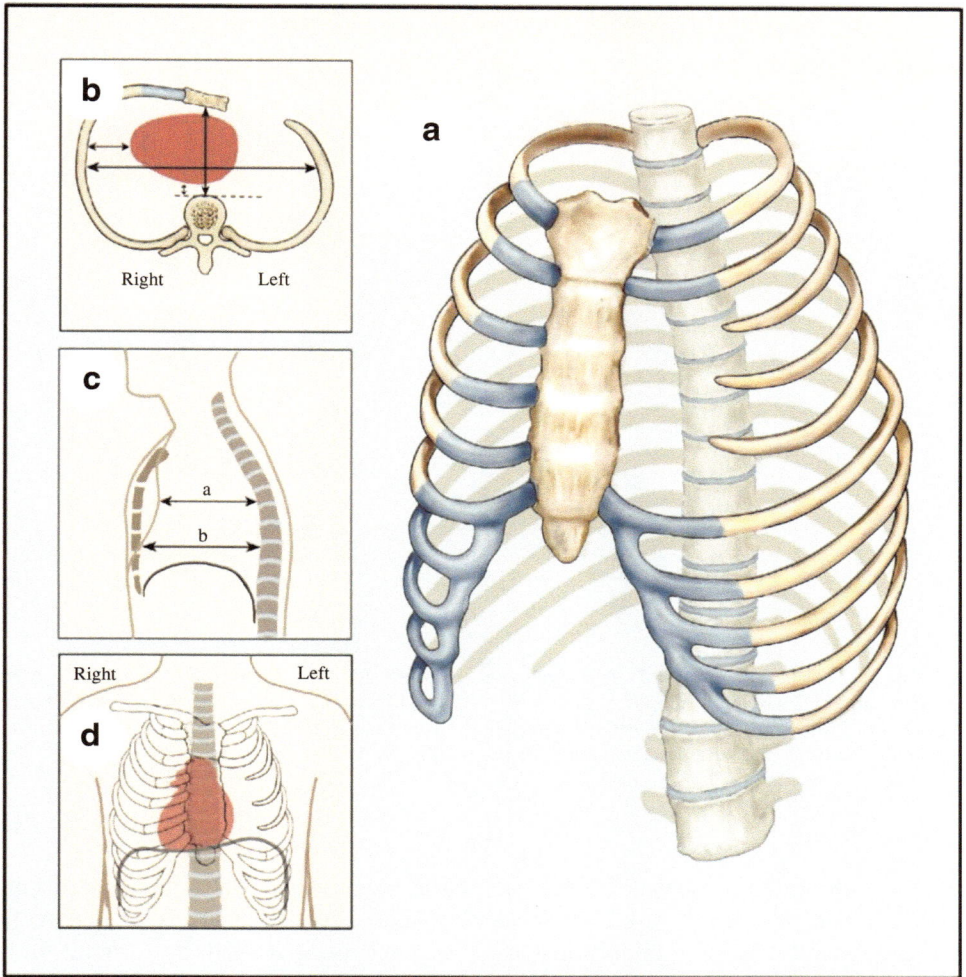

**Fig. 6.4** (**A–D**) Anatomical representation of Poland syndrome. (**A**) Three-dimensional view. Left-sided rib defect. (**B**) Cross-sectional view. Rib defect with chest wall depression and shift of the heart to the right. (**C**) Lateral view. Unilateral chest wall depression. (**D**) Frontal view. Rib defect and isolated dextrocardia. (Used with permission from Fokin, AA.; Steuerwald, NM.; Ahrens, WA.; Allen, KE. Anatomical, Histologic, and Genetic Characteristics of Congenital Chest Wall Deformities. Semin Thorac Cardiovasc Surg. 2009; 21:44–57)

## Diagnosis

Although the presentation of Poland's Syndrome is quite variable, the sine qua none for the disease is the congenital absence of the sternocostal head of the pectoralis major muscle. This reflects the simplest and most common form of the syndrome; and is recognized, in either gender, as an absent anterior axillary fold. The female deformity, in its mildest form, manifests with the concomitant finding of breast hypoplasia. The simultaneous occurrence of additional ipsilateral anomalies of the thorax and upper extremity upstage the diagnosis to one of the more severe forms, rounding out the full spectrum of the syndrome.

Prenatal diagnosis is possible by ultrasonic evaluation; but the diagnosis is more commonly

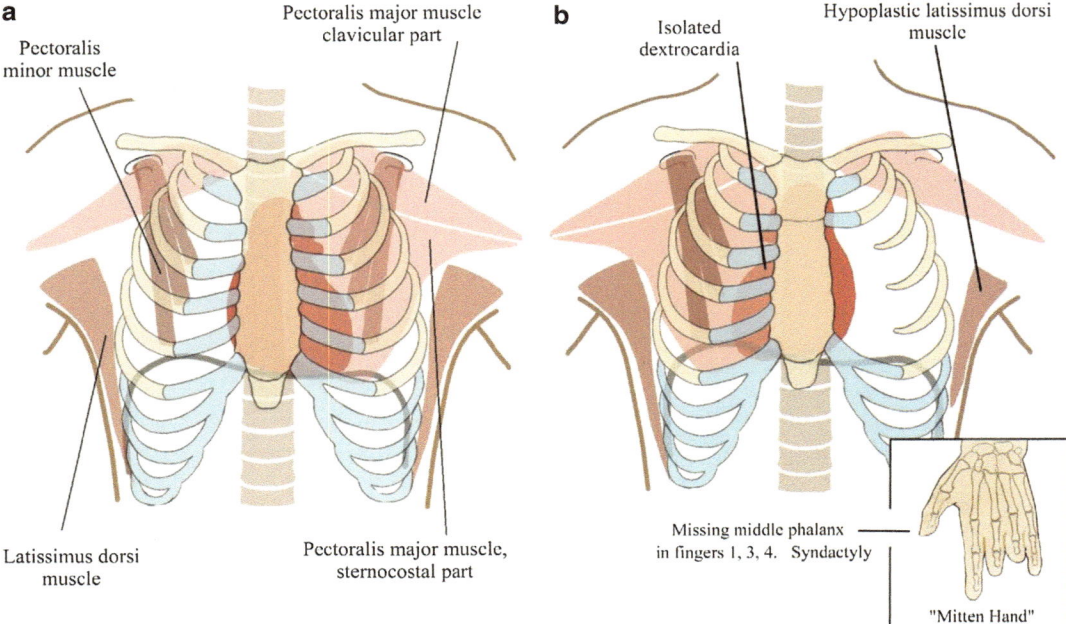

**a**

Pectoralis minor muscle

Pectoralis major muscle clavicular part

Latissimus dorsi muscle

Pectoralis major muscle, sternocostal part

**b**

Isolated dextrocardia

Hypoplastic latissimus dorsi muscle

Missing middle phalanx in fingers 1, 3, 4. Syndactyly

"Mitten Hand"

**Fig. 6.5** (**A**, **B**) Different degrees of Poland syndrome severity. (**A**) Partial PS with pectoral muscle deficit only. (**B**) Full-blown PS with large rib defect, extensive muscle deficit, isolated dextrocardia, and unilateral hand abnormality. (Used with permission from Fokin, AA.; Steuerwald, NM.; Ahrens, WA.; Allen, KE. Anatomical, Histologic, and Genetic Characteristics of Congenital Chest Wall Deformities. Semin Thorac Cardiovasc Surg. 2009; 21:44–57)

made after birth by the constellation of clinical findings [19]. Parents typically notice the severe form of the syndrome early in infancy due to a visibly asymmetric chest wall and brachysyndactyly. The simple form, however, even if known to the patient, may remain hidden from the family until early adolescence when the patient becomes more self-conscious about the asymmetry.

While the majority of patients with Poland's Syndrome present primarily with an aesthetic concern, in the rare case of cardiopulmonary compromise, severe functional impairment is recognized in infancy and should be addressed with prompt surgical intervention. A thorough assessment of *all* patients with Poland's Syndrome is necessary for a complete and accurate diagnosis. Those with the mild form of the syndrome may have measureable differences in the affected hemithorax and upper extremity that may otherwise go unnoticed by visual inspection alone.

This also highlights the importance of a thorough examination in individuals presenting with an apparent isolated syndactyly, as up to 10 % of these patients will have Poland's Syndrome [20].

Physical examination should involve an undraped evaluation of the entire torso and bilateral upper extremities, with inspection, palpation, and measurement of key structural components. This should include measurement of the ribs; as well the distances from sternal notch to acromion, olecranon to ulnar styloid, and lengths of all phalanges; all of which should be compared to measurements on the contralateral, unaffected side. Standard muscle testing is performed, and baseline photographs are taken in the usual fashion [2].

While not a requirement for diagnosis, various imaging modalities may assist with preoperative planning, particularly in cases where autogenous reconstruction is being considered. Computed

Topography (CT), Magnetic Resonance Imaging (MRI), and Angiography are the most useful; permitting a more detailed assessment of the skeletal, soft tissue, and vascular anomalies, respectively. Beer et al., in their report of a case of Poland's Syndrome in a 17-year-old girl, were forced to abort a pedicled latissimus dorsi flap due to severe attenuation of the muscle that was not recognized clinically on preoperative examination. An MRI later confirmed the absence of the latissimus dorsi muscle, with angiography providing the additional findings of subclavian artery hypoplasia and complete absence of its thoracoacromial and thoracodorsal branches. The identification of other coexisting conditions, such as renal agenesis, is another benefit of diagnostic imaging, as this too may affect reconstructive outcomes [15].

## Treatment Considerations

The clinical polymorphism Poland's Syndrome presents with precludes a generalized approach to its surgical management. Rather, an individualized approach is advocated, taking into consideration a number of factors that ultimately influence the therapeutic intervention. The process of arriving at the most appropriate treatment strategy for each patient can be simplified by considering a series of questions provided below:

- *Does the defect present primarily as a functional or aesthetic concern?*
- *Are there significant psychosocial implications affecting this patient at this time?*
- *Has the patient reached skeletal maturity?*
- *What is the gender of the patient?*
- *What is the severity of the syndrome presentation?*

Answers to the first three questions address the issue of *timing of intervention*, while the latter two provide direction with respect to the particular *surgical approach*.

Any surgical intervention on the growing child must be viewed as a balance between the benefit of early correction and the risk of future growth impairment. With the deformities in Poland's Syndrome being predominantly aesthetic in nature, the general consensus is to delay surgical correction until skeletal maturity. Of course, the presence of significant *functional* deformity trumps the risk of early operative intervention. In Poland's Syndrome, severe chest wall deformity causing cardiopulmonary compromise, and syndactyly are two such deformities with significant functional implications that warrant early repair. Another exception, one that addresses an aesthetic issue, is the use of tissue expanders in the hypoplastic breast of the skeletally immature patient. By serially expanding the hypoplastic breast to keep pace with the growing contralateral breast, this can minimize asymmetry and the psychosocial implications accompanying this deformity in the adolescent female patient (Fig. 6.6) [21].

Aside from the few exceptions provided above, surgical correction of Poland's Syndrome is delayed until growth is complete. In individuals who have reached skeletal maturity, the particular surgical approach is influenced by patient gender and syndrome severity. The algorithm for both male and female patients is similar, with the obvious distinction that in the female patient the hypoplastic breast is also addressed. Reconstructive needs in the simple and complex forms of the syndrome differ based upon the nature of the musculoskeletal and soft tissue deficiencies present.

The remainder of this chapter will focus on the surgical management of Poland's Syndrome with a look at the options available for reconstruction of the different forms of the disease. Before we begin, it is worth reviewing the anatomy of the structures typically affected in Poland's Syndrome, paying particular attention to how the aberrations differ from normal anatomy. An understanding of normal anatomy is paramount if one is to restore normal form in these often-complex defects. Ascribing to fundamental reconstructive principles, we shall take an inside-out approach, beginning with a look at thoracic skeleton.

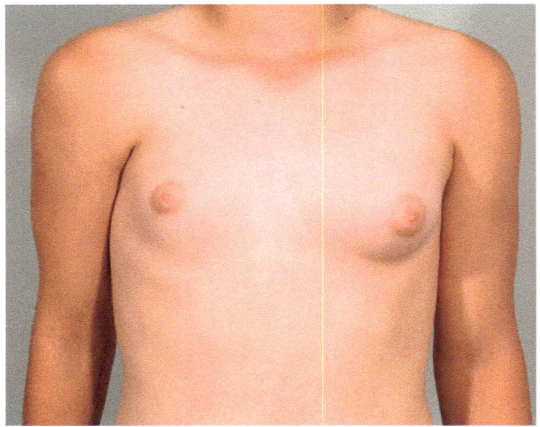 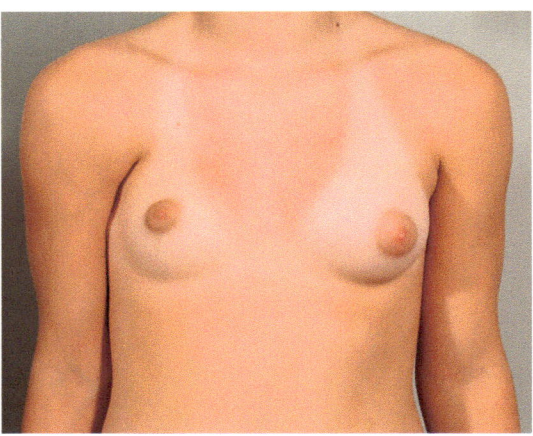

**Fig. 6.6** (*Left*) A 13-year-old girl with mild Poland syndrome. (*Right*) Result after insertion of tissue expander. The plan is to wait until the patient reaches age 17 years to insert a permanent implant. (Used with permission from Pryor, Landon S.; Lehman Jr., James A., Workmann, Meredith C. Disorders of the Female Breast in the Pediatric Age Group. Plast Reconstr Surg. 2009. 126(1S):50e-60e, 2009)

## Anatomy

### Thoracic Skeleton

The normal thoracic skeleton is an osseous cage comprising the sternum, the thoracic vertebrae, 12 pairs of ribs and the clavicles. It houses and protects the heart, lungs, and great vessels of the thorax; serves as a major structural support for the body and upper extremities; and contributes to respiratory function. In the simple (partial or mild) form of Poland's Syndrome, the osseous thorax is entirely normal; the more advanced forms present with rib and sternal aberrations. If these aberrations are severe enough to compromise pulmonary function or protection of the heart, surgical intervention is undertaken early irrespective of skeletal maturity.

Patients with rib and sternal involvement characteristically present with a sunken chest on the affected side (Fig. 6.7). This is caused by hypoplasia of the ribs and cartilages in the moderate form (Fig. 6.8), and aplasia of the anterior portion of the ribs and cartilages in the severe (complete) form of the disease (Fig. 6.9). One to three ribs are

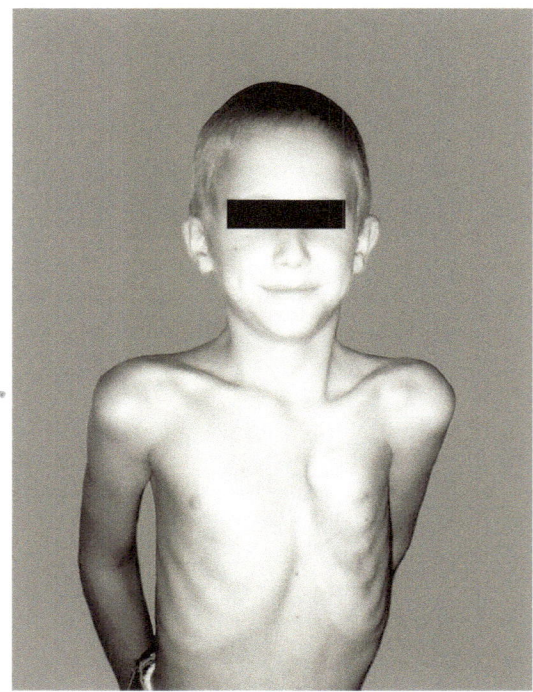

**Fig. 6.7** Photograph of a patient with Poland's syndrome. (Used with permission from Fokin, AA.; Robicsek, F. Poland's Syndrome Revisited. Ann Thorac Surg. 2002; 74:2218–2225)

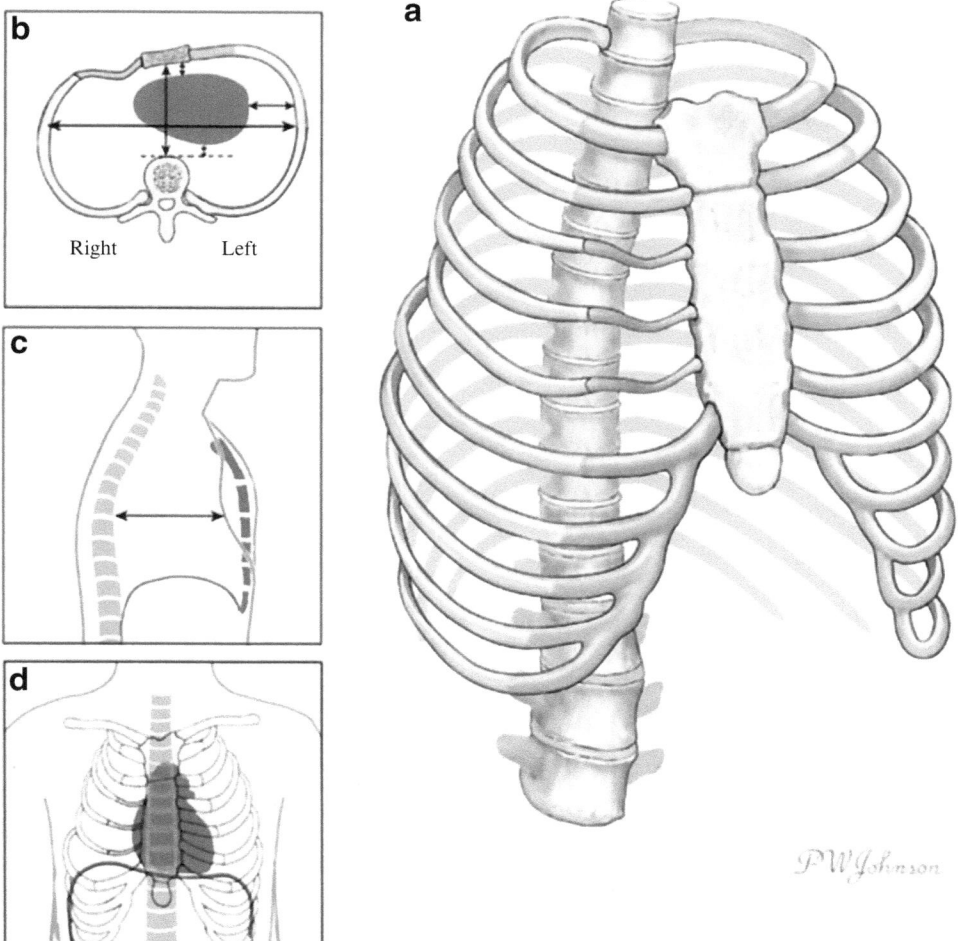

**Fig. 6.8** Chest involvement in moderate form of Poland's syndrome. (**A**) Three-dimensional, oblique view showing chest wall depression with hypoplasia of ribs III to V. Mild rotation of the sternum. (**B**) Cross-sectional view showing normal position of the heart between the sternum and vertebral column. (**C**) Lateral view showing unilateral depression of the ribs. (**D**) Frontal view showing hypoplasia of the involved ribs. Normal position of the heart. (Used with permission from Fokin, AA.; Robicsek, F. Poland's Syndrome Revisited. Ann Thorac Surg. 2002; 74:2218–2225)

typically affected. Ribs 1–3 and ribs 2–4 are the most commonly affected groups, the latter occurring more frequently than the former. In the case of rib aplasia, the sternal ends of the aplastic ribs may be entirely separate or fused together [10].

The sternum is typically rotated to the affected side causing a sunken appearance ipsilaterally and an asymmetrical, contralateral pectus carinatum. In the moderate form, where the thoracic cage remains intact but selectively hypoplastic, the heart maintains its normal position between the sternum and vertebral column. In the severe form, with rib aplasia, the unprotected heart often assumes a more protected position by shifting to the unaffected side. In a series of 144 patients with Poland's Syndrome, the incidence of dextrocardia was noted to be 5.6%. Unlike isolated dextrocardia, which is almost always associated

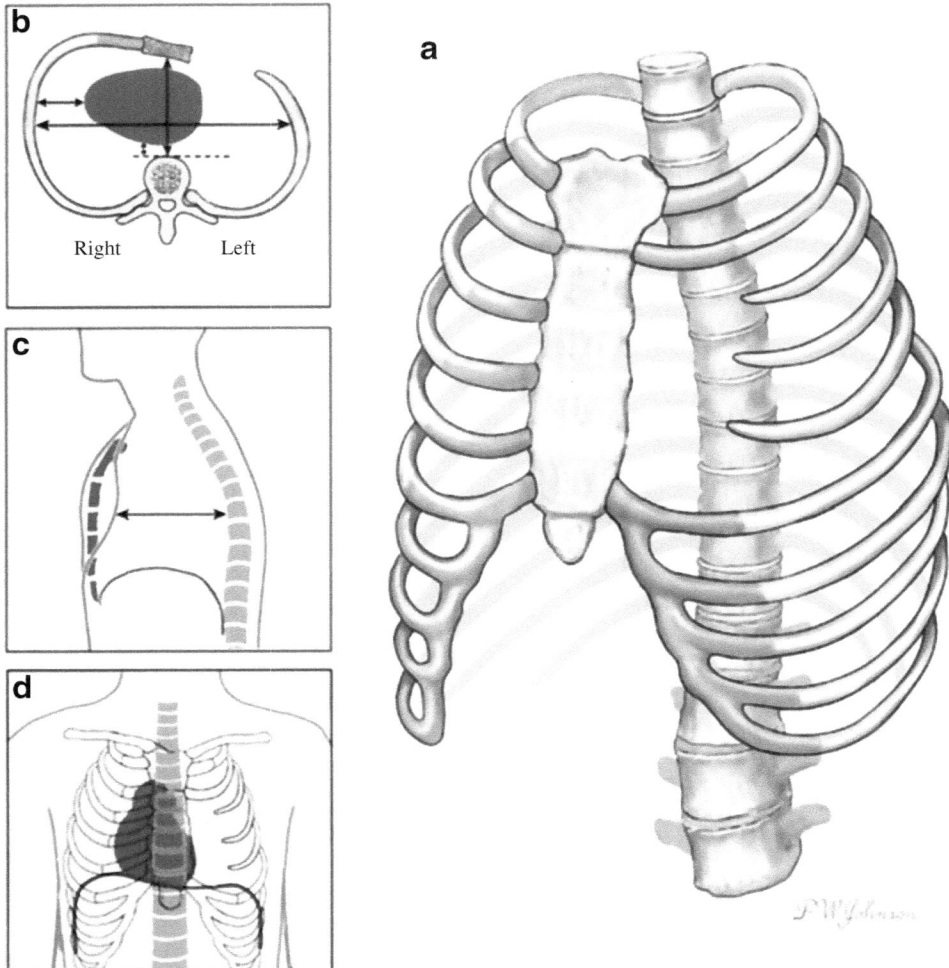

**Fig. 6.9** Chest involvement in severe form of Poland's syndrome. (**A**) Three-dimensional, oblique view showing chest wall defect with aplasia of ribs III to V. Rotation of the sternum. (**B**) Cross-sectional view showing that the unprotected heart is shifted toward the unaffected side. (**C**) Lateral view showing unilateral depression of the ribs. (**D**) Frontal view showing aplasia of the involved ribs. Dextrocardia. (Used with permission from Fokin, AA.; Robicsek, F. Poland's Syndrome Revisited. Ann Thorac Surg. 2002; 74:2218–2225

with other cardiovascular anomalies, dextrocardia in Poland's Syndrome is not [10].

The lack of an intact thoracic cage can also manifest as lung herniation with paradoxical motion of the chest wall. This can reduce vital capacity thereby compromising respiratory function. The incidence of lung herniation is reported to be 8 % [10].

## Muscles of the Chest Wall

The thoracic skeleton is covered by muscle, subcutaneous tissue, and skin. Those muscles with their origin and/or insertion on the bony thorax serve one of two main functions: (1) to facilitate respiration and (2) to serve as a means of attachment for and support the upper extremities. The muscle invariably affected in all forms of the disease is the pectoralis major muscle. The pectoralis minor muscle is often affected as well; and variable deformities of the serratus, infraspinatus, supraspinatus, latissimus dorsi, and external oblique muscles can also be seen. These are all stabilization muscles, none of which have any respiratory function. Furthermore, the deformities in these muscles, when present, fail to result in any significant functional impairment, even from an upper extremity perspective.

The main muscular deformity deserving surgical consideration is the absence of the sternocostal head of the pectoralis major muscle. The pectoralis major is a large, fan-shaped muscle covering much of the anterior chest wall divided into three portions, each with an independent origin but with a common insertion on the humerus.

The clavicular head is the most cephalad, and it arises from the medial third of the clavicle. The central portion, or sternocostal head, is the largest having a broad origin along the sternum and the costal cartilages of the first six ribs. The third origin, from the external oblique aponeurosis, is variable in size. The fibers from all origins converge to form a common tendon that passes deep to the deltoid muscle to insert on to the greater tuberosity of the humerus. In doing so, it forms the anterior axillary fold.

The large, fan-shaped sternocostal head of the pectoralis major muscle is invariably absent in all forms of the disease and is pathognomonic for Poland's Syndrome. This renders the ipsilateral anterior axillary fold (formed by the inferior border of the sternocostal head) deficient. With the absence of a well-defined anterior axillary fold, the posterior axillary fold (formed by the latissimus dorsi and teres major muscles) can be seen from the front. This presents as an obvious asymmetry readily noticed and remarked upon by the patient. Absence of the sternocostal head of the pectoralis major muscle also creates an accentuated infraclavicular hollow that adds to the asymmetry. This, along with the deficient anterior axillary fold, must be addressed if an acceptable reconstructive outcome is to be expected.

The pectoralis minor is seen as a thin triangular bundle attaching the humerus to the inferomedial third of the clavicle. It may be diminutive, particular in the complex form. Again in the complex form, an axillary web may be seen, which may seemingly contain muscular tissue as it can appear to have contractile activity [2, 15]. The serratus anterior may also be absent, causing a winging of the scapula.

## Breast

The adult breast extends from the second to seventh rib in the mid clavicular line and from the sternocostal junction medially to the midaxillary line laterally. The inframammary fold forms the inferior border of the breast, and it is a distinct anatomic structure representing the fusion of the deep and superficial fascia with the dermis of the skin. The fibers of the inframammary fold are arranged in a crisscross fashion, anchoring the skin in place and forming a stable inferior border for the otherwise pendulous breast.

The upper pole of the breast is less full than the lower pole. When viewed in profile, the outer contour of the upper pole should be seen as a smooth and even slope from the clavicle to the nipple-areolar-complex. The outer contour of the lower pole, rather, with its increased fullness, has a gentle curvature from the nipple-areolar-complex to the inframammary fold. The nipple-areolar-complex is ideally centered over the greatest prominence of the breast mound, placing it at the junction of the upper and lower poles and mediolaterally in the midclavicular line. In idealistic proportions, if an equilateral triangle is drawn with its apex at the sternal notch, the right and left corners of the base of this triangle will be centered precisely over the right and left nipples, respectively.

In Poland's Syndrome, breast involvement in the female patient varies from mild hypoplasia to complete absence (amastia). The nipple-areolar-complex is likewise hypoplastic. It is typically elevated and hypopigmented, and occasionally even completely absent (athelia). With respect to positioning, it appears displaced towards the axilla, being somewhat more superiorly and laterally positioned than its contralateral counterpart.

## Surgical Management

The main goals of surgical correction in Poland's Syndrome are to improve chest wall symmetry and, in the female patient, to correct breast hypoplasia or asymmetry. Creation of an anterior axillary fold and softening of the infraclavicular hollow are of paramount importance in achieving an excellent result. To provide the best symmetry, any underlying skeletal deformity must also be addressed to provide a solid uniform base for overlying soft tissue reconstruction.

As previously mentioned, severe aplasia causing a compromise in pulmonary function or protection of the heart warrants early surgical correction. These cases are performed in stages, with the skeletal reconstruction occurring in childhood and the soft tissue (muscle +/− breast) reconstruction postponed until after puberty. The correction of skeletal aberrations *without* functional implication is often performed in a delayed, single-stage, multi-layered fashion once growth is complete.

## Skeletal Reconstruction

The reconstructive approach to the thoracic skeleton in Poland's Syndrome evolved as a corollary from the surgical correction of Pectus Excavatum.

In the arena of corrective surgery for depressive chest wall deformities, the procedure that has gained the most recognition over the past half century or so is the Ravitch Procedure. First described by Mark Ravitch in 1949, the procedure entailed the resection of all deformed costal cartilages, a sternal wedge osteotomy, and division of the xiphi-sternal articulation and substernal ligament. The objective was to completely free the sternum of all restriction prior to repositioning it in its corrected position [22, 23].

In 1965, Ravitch revised his original procedure in an effort to achieve a more effective elevation of the sternum and prevent recurrence. To do so, he used an interpositional bone graft at the sternal osteotomy site and oblique chondrotomies with overlap fixation at the second or third costal cartilages. His "revised" procedure is what is commonly referred to today as the "Ravitch Procedure" [24].

Further modifications were made by Haller and Fonkalsrud. Concerned with the longevity of the reconstructive outcome, Haller advocated for the placement of a temporary stainless steel strut beneath the sternum, removing it 6–9 months later as a secondary procedure. Believing that too early and too extensive of an operation on a young child could lead to restriction of future chest growth, he shortened the length of cartilage resection, and delayed any operative intervention until after 4 years of age [25, 26]. In keeping with Haller's less invasive approach, Fonkalsrud followed suit with his modification of the Ravitch Procedure. Noting that the regenerated costal cartilages (after radical resection) were thin, irregular, and rigid with calcification, the "Fonkalsrud Procedure" removed only short 3–8 mm segments of cartilage from both the medial and the lateral ends. The large intervening segments of cartilage that remained were then reattached to the sternum and the ribs. A transverse sternal wedge osteotomy and placement of a stainless steel Adkins strut were used to elevate and secure the sternum in its corrected position; the Adkins strut was then removed in a second-stage procedure [27]. The Haller and Fonkalsrud modifications (and any other variations) are what are referred to today as "modified Ravitch" procedures.

In contrast to open techniques, Nuss, in 1998, described his minimally invasive approach [28]. The Nuss procedure corrects the thoracic cage deformity with a retrosternal metal bar without the use of large incisions or resection of costal cartilages. The procedure involves slipping in one or more concave steel bars into the chest deep to the sternum, and then flipping the bar to a convex position. The twisting of the bar into the convex position pushes the depressed sternum outward, thereby correcting the deformity. The bar typically remains in place for 2–5 years until its removal as an outpatient procedure. The merits of this procedure are in its minimally invasive approach; however, recurrence rates tend to be higher than with open repair, and its utility may be limited in the more severe cases.

In Poland's Syndrome, the thoracic skeletal deformity can be thought of as an ipsilateral pectus excavatum with a contralateral pectus carinatum. The unilateral aplasia/hypoplasia of the costal cartilages causes a rotation of the sternum to the affected side thereby resulting in a depression-type deformity ipsilaterally and a concomitant protrusion-type deformity contralaterally. With its resection of costal cartilages and sternal repositioning, the Ravitch procedure (or one of its variations) has proven effective at addressing both deformities and has traditionally served as the benchmark procedure for surgical management of thoracic skeletal deformity in Poland's Syndrome (Fig. 6.10).

Recall, however, that not all patients with Poland's Syndrome present with thoracic skeletal aberrations. In the "simple" form of Poland's Syndrome, only the soft tissues are affected; the thoracic skeleton is intact and completely normal. It is only in the "moderate" (rib hypoplasia) and "severe" (rib aplasia) forms that the option of skeletal reconstruction is entertained (Fig. 6.11).

Do all patients with thoracic skeletal deformity require reconstruction? Clearly no, as the decision to proceed with reconstruction depends on severity of the deformity, patient desires, and surgeon goals. In Shamberger's series of 75 patients with Poland's Syndrome, 51 patients had either a completely normal chest wall or some evidence of rib hypoplasia *without* contour deformity. The remaining 24 patients presented with either a depression deformity (16 patients) or rib aplasia (8 patients). Only ten of these patients required reconstruction. Seven of the ten patients underwent surgery to correct a significantly rotated sternum and contralateral carinate deformity; only three patients received rib grafts for rib aplasia. In this series, of the 24 patients that had a thoracic deformity, less than half were

deemed substantial enough to warrant surgical intervention. The authors conclude that all patients with absent ribs and all patients with severe ipsilateral concave deformity should be considered candidates for repair, with the vital components of the repair being correction of the abnormally positioned and rotated sternum and replacement of the absent ribs [29]. Haller emphasizes the importance of rib grafts in cases of rib aplasia not only for chest wall stability to achieve a sound base for further reconstruction, but to prevent potential lung herniation. While not typically present in the young child, lung herniation can become a severe physiological problem later on in life once the child enters teenage years or young adulthood [30].

Rib aplasia can be addressed with autologous rib grafts, as in the original Ravitch Procedure; autologous soft tissue in the form of vascularized muscle flaps; foreign material in the form of various meshes or implants; or a combination of methods (Fig. 6.12). Ipsilateral or contralateral autologous rib grafts can be used depending on which ribs are affected. In the original Ravitch procedure, a woven Dacron fabric was used in addition to autologous rib grafts to replace the missing endothoracic fascia and add stability to the reconstruction. Haller et al., concerned with the use of a large foreign body in the growing child, combined the use of an ipsilateral, pedicled latissimus dorsi muscle flap with the basic structural reconstruction of the Ravitch chest wall repair to achieve chest wall stabilization and immediate aesthetic reconstruction without prostheses. The majority of patients in their series were male patients, all except one, and therefore did not require breast reconstruction (Fig. 6.13) [30]. A well-illustrated example of a similar procedure can be seen in Seyfer's 2010 review of 63 patients with Poland's Syndrome [2].

In the female patient desiring breast reconstruction, a single-stage procedure combining skeletal, muscle, and breast reconstruction is preferred. In the patient with an intact and normal thoracic cage, a breast prosthesis with a latissimus dorsi muscle flap is frequently employed to create an anterior axillary fold and enhance soft

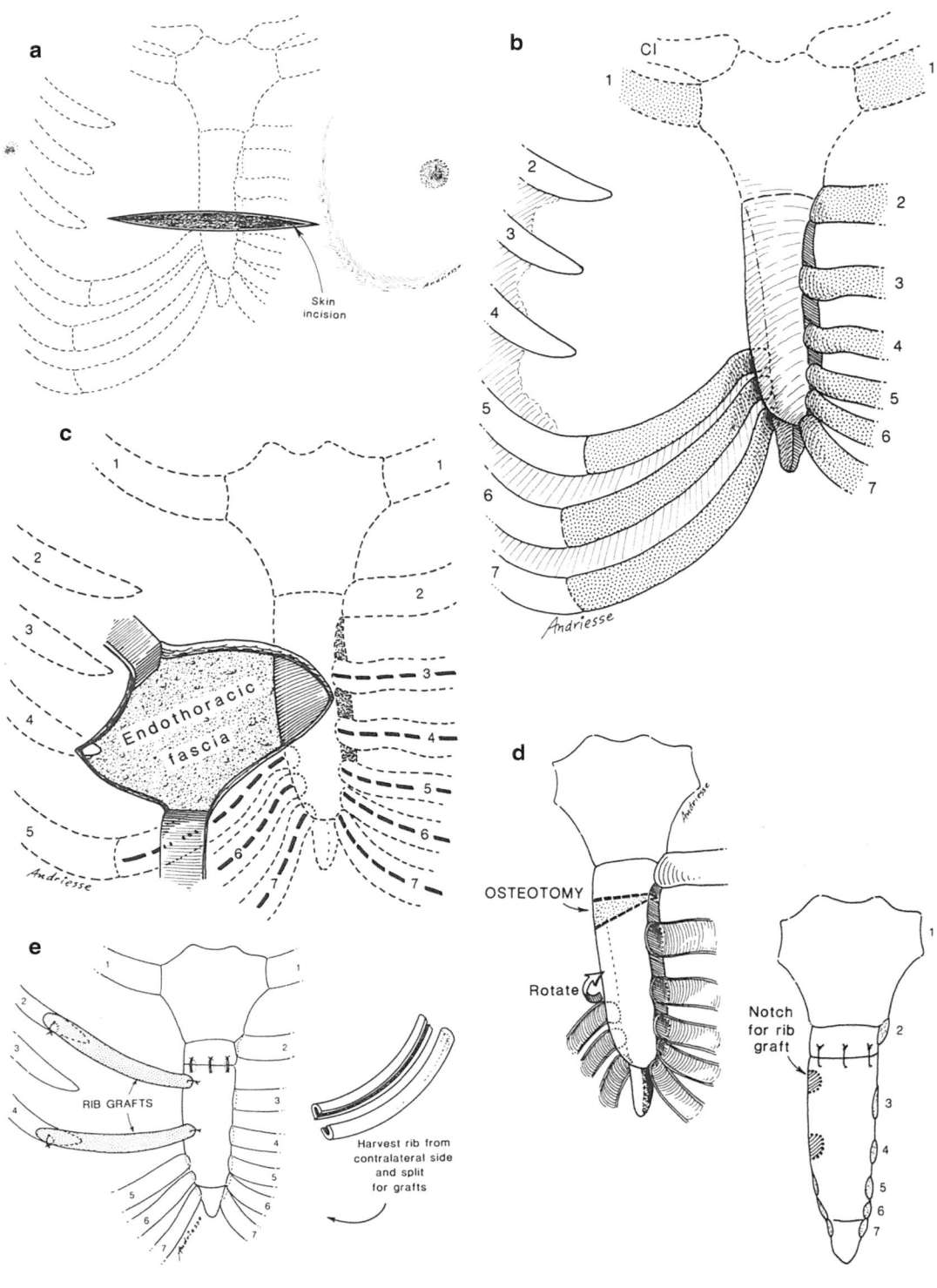

a Skin incision

b Cl

c Endothoracic fascia

d OSTEOTOMY

Rotate

Notch for rib graft

e RIB GRAFTS

Harvest rib from contralateral side and split for grafts

tissue fill in the region. In cases of rib aplasia, if the latissimus muscle is used in the base layer reconstruction, as Haller described, it would be unavailable for coverage over the breast prosthesis, and the reconstruction may fail to address the issue of the infraclavicular hollow. Fokin and Robicsek advocate rib grafts and/or mesh to address the aplastic rib defect and concomitant myocutaneous latissimus dorsi flap and breast

prosthesis to correct the muscle deficiency and breast hypoplasia, respectively (Fig. 6.14).

For skeletal chest wall deformities not reaching the level where Ravitch or Nuss procedures are being considered, these aesthetic deformities can be managed by implants to restore continuity and/or improve contour. Synthetic, biologic, and autologous can be used to address concavities secondary to less severe skeletal abnormalities or

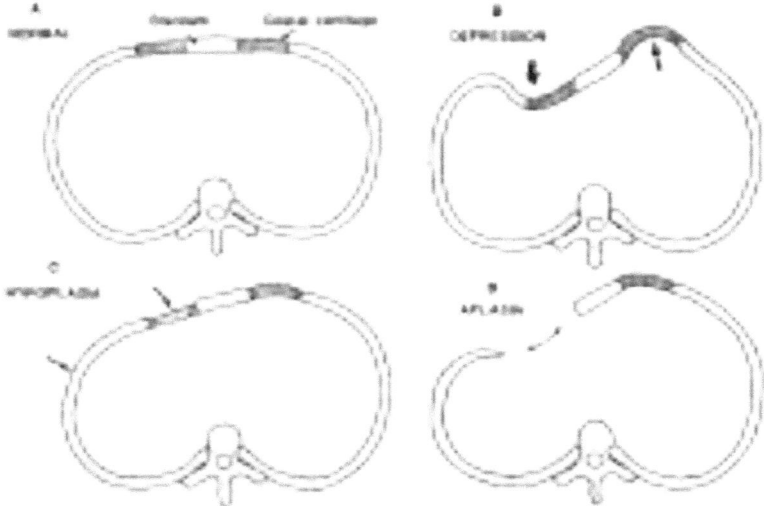

**Fig. 6.11** The spectrum of rib cage abnormality seen in Poland's Syndrome is shown. (**A**) Most frequently an entirely normal rib cage is seen with only the pectoral muscles absent. (**B**) Depression of the involved side of the chest wall with rotation and often depression of the sternum. A carinate protrusion of the contralateral side is frequently present. (**C**) Hypoplasia of the ribs on the involved side but without significant depression might be seen. (**D**) Aplasia of one or more ribs is usually associated with depression of adjacent ribs on the involved side and rotation of the sternum. (Used with permission from Shamberger, RC., Welch, KJ., Upton III, J. Surgical treatment of thoracic deformity in Poland's syndrome. J Pediatr Surg. 1989; 24(8): 760-766)

**Fig. 6.10** (**A**) A transverse incision is placed below the nipple line and in females at the site of the future inframammary crease. (**B**) Schematic depiction of the deformity with rotation of the sternum, depression of the cartiages of the involved side, and carinate protrusion of the contralateral side. (**C**) In cases with aplasia of the ribs, the endothoracic fascia is encountered directly below the attenuated subcutaneous tissue and pectoral fascia. The pectoral muscle flap is elevated on the contralateral side and the pectoral fascia, if present, on the involved side. Subperichondrial resection of the costal cartilages is carried out as shown by the dashed lines. Rarely, this must be carried to the level of the second costal cartilage. (**D**) A transverse offset wedge-shaped sternal osteotomy is then created below the second costal cartilage. Closure of the defect with heavy silk sutures corrects both the posterior displacement and the rotation of the sternum. (**E**) In cases with rib aplasia, split rib grafts are harvested from the contralateral fifth or sixth ribs and then secured medially with wire sutures into previously created sternal notched and with wire to the native ribs laterally. Ribs are split as shown along their short axis to maintain maximum mechanical strength. (Used with permission from Shamberger, RC., Welch, KJ., Upton III, J. Surgical treatment of thoracic deformity in Poland's syndrome. J Pediatr Surg. 1989; 24(8): 760–766)

**a**

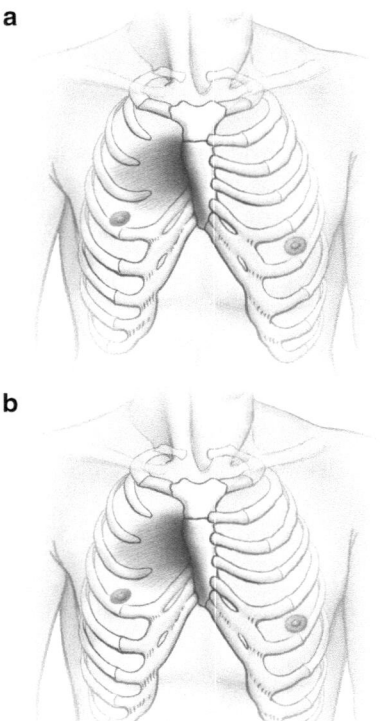

**b**

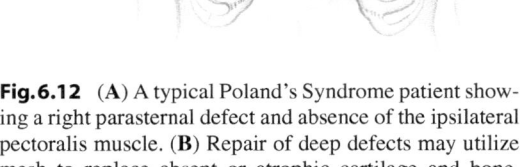

**c**

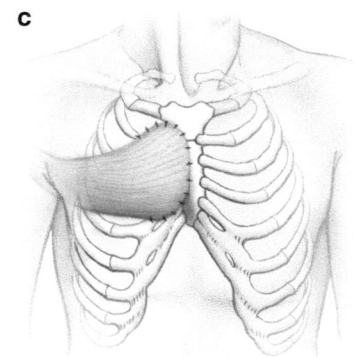

**Fig. 6.12** (**A**) A typical Poland's Syndrome patient show-ing a right parasternal defect and absence of the ipsilateral pectoralis muscle. (**B**) Repair of deep defects may utilize mesh to replace absent or atrophic cartilage and bone.

(**C**) A latissimus dorsi muscle flap recreates the anterior axillary fold and corrects soft tissue symmetry. (Used with permission from Moir, CR.; Johnson, CH. Poland's syndrome. Semin Pediatr Surg. 2008; 17: 161–166)

residual deformities following Nuss or Ravitch procedures.

Soft, silicone gel prostheses have been com-monly used to address thoracic contour defor-mity in Poland's Syndrome and are available as either custom-made or prefabricated options. The appeal in their use is in the much shorter and less invasive operative procedure compared to autol-ogous options, with less morbidity and a more rapid patient recovery. Unfortunately, complica-tions, such as implant slippage or displacement, residual contour irregularities, and discomfort are not uncommon. Extrusion is also a concern when using an implant; thus, adequate soft tissue coverage is of paramount importance. This could not be more relevant than in Poland's Syndrome, where the pectoralis major muscle is absent and

the overlying skin and subcutaneous tissues are thin and deficient. A soft, silicone prosthesis has the advantage, therefore, of exerting less pressure on the deficient overlying soft tissues. A more solid material (e.g. methyl methacrylate), in con-trast, would offer the additional benefit of improved stability, albeit at the potential cost of a more substantial soft tissue cover requirement.

Synthetic patches or meshes have been used for decades with excellent results in stabilization of a variety of chest wall defects, including those from Poland's Syndrome. A number exist, each with product-specific advantages and disadvantages. As with any synthetic implant, the primary benefit is the lack of donor site morbidity. Drawbacks, however, are an often-incomplete incorporation, susceptibility to infection necessitating implant

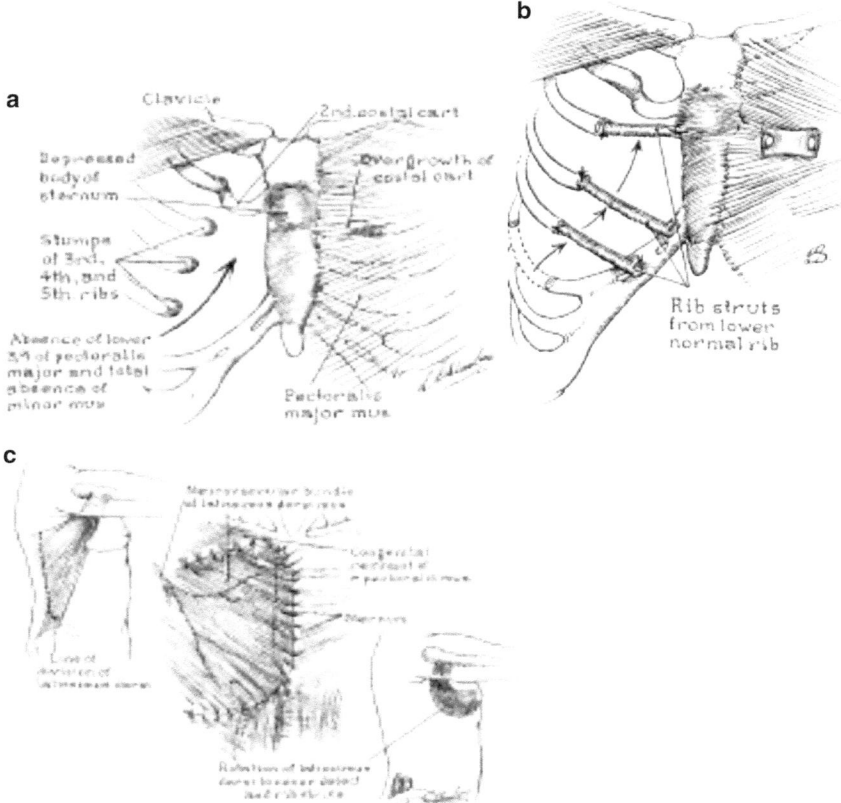

**Fig. 6.13** (**A**) Anatomy of Right Poland's Syndrome with missing cartilage of ribs 3, 4, & 5 and rotation of the sternum. (**B**) Autologous rib strut from rib 6, resection of overgrowth of left rib cartilage 3. (**C**) Rotation of Latissimus dorsi muscle flap to augment soft tissue defect and protect chest wall reconstruction. (Used with permission from Haller Jr., AJ.; Colombani, PM.; Miller, D; Manson, P. Early reconstruction of Poland's syndrome using autologous rib grafts combined with a latissimus muscle flap. J Pediatr Surg. 1984; 19(4): 423–429)

removal, and adhesion formation with the potential for visceral injury. These limitations are not infrequently encountered, particularly in complex and/or contaminated wounds.

Bioprosthetics have evolved precisely to circumvent these issues. Acellular dermal matrices (ADM) are created from full-thickness sections of human cadaveric, porcine, or bovine skin that is subsequently decellularized to remove antigenic material. The inflammatory response after implantation is mitigated in comparison to synthetic materials; and it shows rapid cellular infiltration, vascularization, and good incorporation in tissue, favoring its use in more hostile wound environments. If infection does occur,

ADM has the added benefit of not requiring removal. Rather, a more conservative approach is adopted with antibiotics and local wound care being the mainstay of management. Seroma formation and the increased cost of ADM (relative to synthetic alternatives) are the main disadvantages.

## Soft Tissue Reconstruction

In the case of the male patient with Poland's Syndrome, the goals of soft tissue reconstruction are to create symmetry of the soft tissue chest by restoring contour deficits and re-creating the

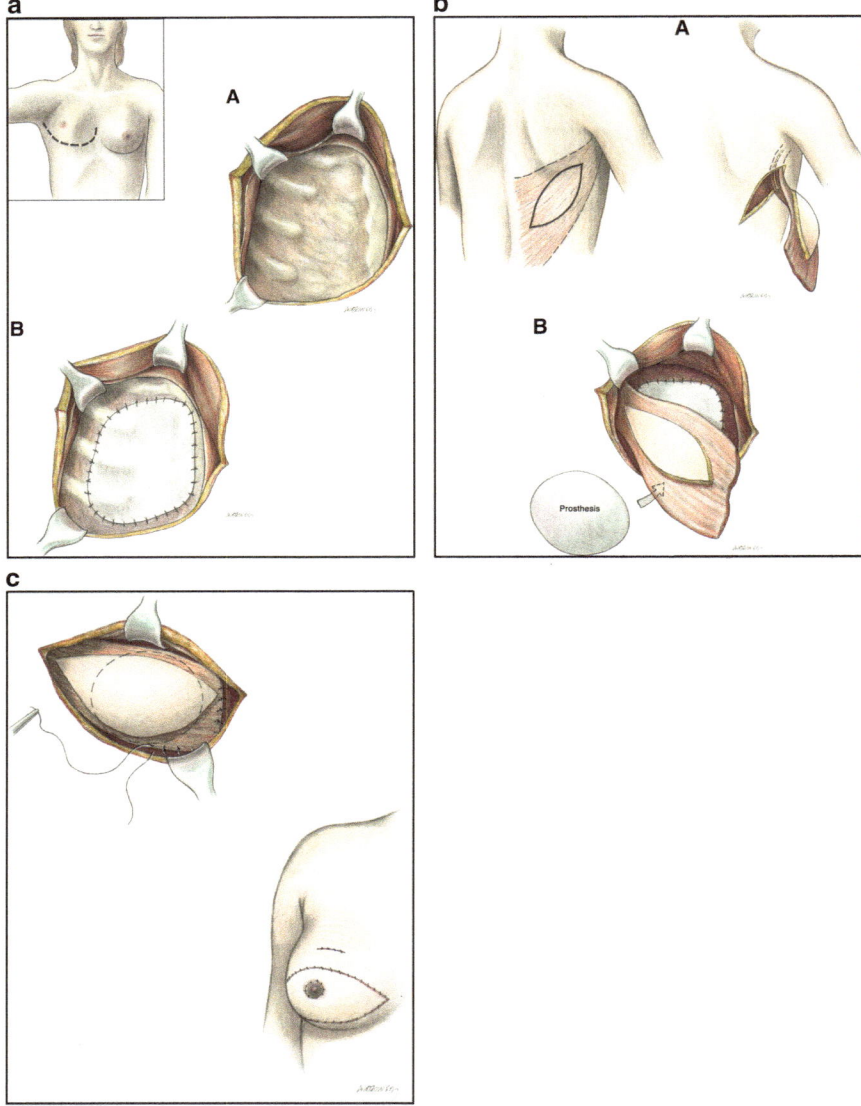

**Fig. 6.14** Single-stage chest wall and breast reconstruction in the female patient with Poland's Syndrome. (Used with permission from Urschel Jr., HC. Poland syndrome. Semin Thorac Cardiovasc Surg. 2009; 21(1): 89–94)

absent anterior axillary fold. In the female patient, the goals are similar with the additional objective of creating a symmetrical breast. In either gender, a number of reconstructive options exist and they include the following:

- Implant alone
- Implant with flap
- Flap alone
- Autologous fat grafting

## Implant Alone

Implants alone have been used in select cases of Poland's Syndrome. Their use is most suited for male patients with the "simple" or "mild" form of the syndrome, where only soft tissue deficits exist. Most pectoral implants used for this purpose are made of a soft, cohesive silicone gel; and are available as custom made or prefabricated prostheses. The appeal is a much shorter and less invasive operative procedure and a more rapid patient recovery.

A number of complications, however, have been reported. These include the typical implant complications of infection, hematoma, seroma, capsule formation, displacement, and extrusion. Implant extrusion is a particular concern in Poland's Syndrome, where the overlying soft tissues are inherently thin or deficient.

In the female patient with Poland's Syndrome, use of an implant alone to correct a hypoplastic breast deformity may be selected for mild cases. This approach, however, is problematic in the more severe deformities, as it fails to address the absent anterior axillary fold, and does not provide the often-needed soft tissue coverage for the implant. Additionally, augmentation of the breast alone, without adjunctive techniques, accentuates the infraclavicular hollow. Use of autologous fat grafting can be combined with implant-based reconstruction to soften the infraclavicular region and create the appearance of an anterior axillary fold.

While Implant-based breast reconstruction may be performed in a single stage in select cases, a staged approach with an initial insertion of a tissue expander, followed by expander exchange for the final prosthesis after an intermediary period of tissue expansion can be especially useful in the treatment of Poland's Syndrome patients. With this approach, the creation of a precisely positioned inframammary fold, often absent in Poland's Syndrome patients and critical to a successful reconstructive outcome, may be created. By securing an ADM to the chest wall at the level of the desired neo-inframmary fold, an "internal sling" is created to support and properly position the prosthesis. ADM also has the additional benefit of providing an additional layer over the prosthesis, which can be particularly helpful in cases where soft tissue coverage is scarce, as in Poland's Syndrome. Of note, however, the additional volume gained by incorporating ADM into the reconstruction is negligible; and does not negate this shortcoming of the "implant-alone" approach.

## Implant with Flap

To recreate an anterior axillary fold and provide fill of the infraclavicular region, the "implant with flap" approach has traditionally been used for female patients with Poland's Syndrome. The pedicled latissimus dorsi muscle is typically harvested as a myocutaneous flap, as the added soft tissue of the skin paddle provides further volume for augmentation and skin cover for the prosthesis. By disinserting the muscle from the humerus and reattaching it in a more anterior position, an anterior axillary fold is created. The ipsilateral latissimus, however, is occasionally affected and may be found to be deficient or even completely absent. A contralateral free myocutaneous latissimus dorsi flap may be considered in these cases.

Despite its frequent use and consistent results, the latissimus dorsi flap does have disadvantages. Used for reconstruction of what is primarily an aesthetic deformity, the latissimus dorsi flap can leave a long and unsightly donor site scar. Endoscopic approaches have been used to minimize incisions; however, all approaches (endoscopic or open) inevitably create a donor site deformity seen as a deficient posterior axillary fold. Finally, the loss of muscle function must be considered in all cases of muscle transfer; further contributing to the donor site morbidity experienced with latissimus dorsi muscle transfer.

An alternative flap consideration for use in implant-based reconstructions is the omental flap. Effective at creating the anterior axillary fold and obliterating the infraclavicular hollow, the pedicled omental flap can also be harvested laparoscopically to minimize donor site scar. While there is minimal donor site morbidity, it does carry with it all the typical risks of a laparoscopic procedure.

## Flap Alone

The "flap alone" approach can be used in both the male and female patient with Poland's Syndrome. This approach avoids any implant-associated complications. The reconstruction is completely autologous, appearing more natural to the eye and feeling more natural to the touch, with the added benefit of improved longevity of the reconstructive outcome.

The choice of flap for "flap only" reconstructions differs depending on gender of the patient.

For the male patient, the most frequently used flap is the ipsilateral latissimus dorsi muscle flap. It fulfills the objectives of male soft tissue chest wall reconstruction by creating an anterior axillary fold and filling the contour deformity; and it does so with a relatively simple, pedicled approach. Unlike in the female patient, where added tissue bulk is desired, in the male patient the flap is more commonly harvested as a muscle-only flap. The myocutaneous option, however, may also be of benefit in the male patient, particularly in cases of mild skeletal chest wall depression.

While the ipsilateral pedicled latissimus flap is frequently used, other flaps may be chosen to avoid the morbidity associated with latissimus muscle harvest. A free anterolateral thigh (ALT) dermo-adiposal perforator flap can be used to create a well-defined anterior axillary fold and to address chest contour deformity. As this flap contains no muscle, there is no associated loss of muscle function with its use.

Similarly, a transverse musculocutaneous gracilis flap can be used to address the anterior axillary fold and infraclavicular region. Designed correctly, there is little visible scarring and insignificant donor weakness associated with using this small muscle.

While the latissimus flap is the workhorse for male Poland's Syndrome patients, it does not provide enough soft tissue volume to address both the contour deformity of the chest wall and the hypoplastic breast in the female patient. If a pedicled latissimus or omental flap is chosen, augmentation with an implant is typically required. If the patient desires an entirely autologous breast reconstruction, abdominally based flaps are often selected to provide the needed volume.

Since its inception in the late 1970s, the workhorse for autologous breast reconstruction has been the transverse rectus abdominus myocutaneous (TRAM) flap. With more emphasis being placed on minimizing donor site morbidity, free TRAMs and muscle-sparing perforator flap alternatives have become increasingly popular. Although a number of perforator flaps have been described, the abdomen remains the preferred tissue source for breast reconstruction with the deep inferior epigastric artery perforator (DIEP) flap typically being the flap of choice. Additionally, if patient anatomy permits, a superficial inferior epigastric artery (SIEA) flap can also be used.

While the DIEP flap and other abdominally based flaps have been used for autologous breast and chest wall reconstruction in Poland's Syndrome, not all patients with Poland's Syndrome are candidates for abdominally based flaps. Unlike their post-mastectomy counterparts, patients with Poland's Syndrome are typically younger and thinner and may not have adequate abdominal soft tissue excess to support a DIEP or TRAM flap of sufficient bulk. When the abdomen has insufficient volume for breast reconstruction, an assessment of other donor areas is necessary.

The buttocks can serve as a comparable donor site. Basing the flap on the superior or inferior gluteal arteries, a superior gluteal artery perforator (SGAP) or inferior gluteal artery perforator (IGAP) flap can be harvested. Although not a perforator flap, the transverse myocutaneous gracilis (TMG) flap should be considered and has been advocated for as a first-line option. Unilateral or bilateral TMG flaps can be used for independent or simultaneous breast and chest wall reconstruction in the female Poland's Syndrome patient. Donor site morbidity is low and donor site scar is inconspicuous. The thoracodorsal artery perforator (TDAP) flap is another option. It is the perforator flap alternative to the latissimus flap. Sparing the muscle, the donor site morbidity of the TDAP flap is superior to that of the latissimus flap; however, the donor site scar is still more objectionable than that of either the DIEP or gluteal artery flap alternatives, and often it does not have sufficient volume to reconstruct the breast. Finally, a fasciocutaneous ALT flap is yet another perforator flap option that may be considered. Tissue bulk, however, may be a problem in the thin patient; and the donor site scar is not inconspicuous.

## Autologous Fat Grafting

Introduced by Illouz in 1986 and comprehensively detailed by Coleman nearly a decade later, the injection of autologous fat has emerged as a viable and ever-promising technique to address a variety of defects ranging from small contour irregularities to complete breast reconstruction. Also termed lipofilling or lipomodelling, it offers the advantage of using autologous tissue, with limited scarring and donor site morbidity. Not only does it provide volume, it has the added benefit of inducing positive change in the recipient tissues, yielding a softer and more supple result.

In the context of chest wall reconstruction in Poland's Syndrome, autologous fat injection appears to be particularly useful in filling the infraclavicular hollow and providing volume for restoration of the deficient anterior axillary fold. Pinsolle et al. report their experience using autologous fat injection in patients with Poland's Syndrome. In their small series of eight patients (seven women, one man), lipofilling was used most often as an adjunctive technique to provide additional volume and to improve contour not addressed by conventional techniques alone (Fig. 6.15).

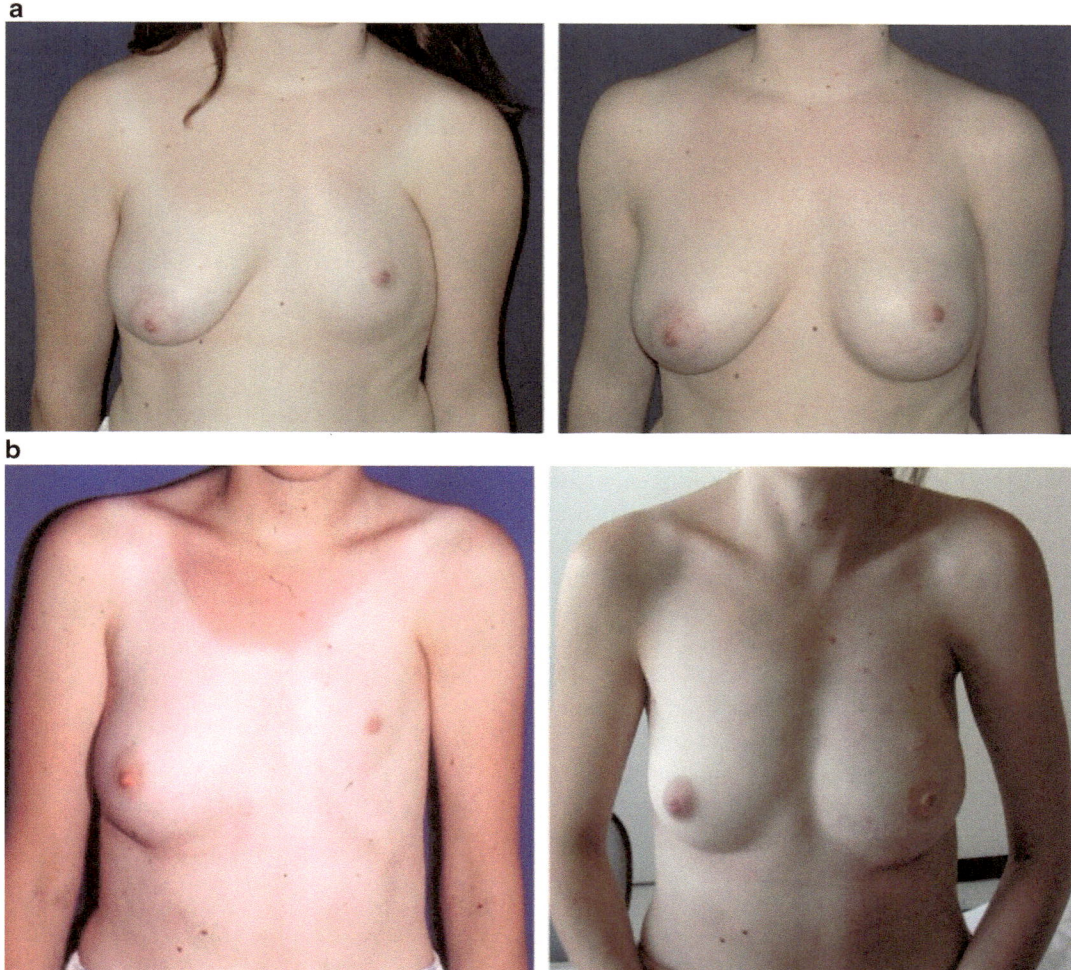

**Fig. 6.15** (**A**) 17-year-old woman treated with a breast implant after skin expansion and two sessions of fat injection to fill the anterior axillary fold and the subclavicular hollow. Left: preoperative view. Right: postoperative result at 16 months. (**B**) 20-year-old woman treated with a latissimus dorsi flap, a breast implant after skin expansion, a customized silicone implant and one session of fat injection to fill the anterior axillary fold. Left: preoperative view. Right: postoperative result at 1 year. (Used with permission from Pinsolle, V.; Chichery, A.; Grolleau, J-L.; Chavoin, JP. Autologous fat injection in Poland's syndrome. J Plast Reconstr Aesthet Surg. 2008; 61:784–791

Autologous fat injection has also proven effective in breast reconstruction; not only as an adjunctive procedure, but as a sole modality of treatment. Delay et al. in their 2010 report of an 11-year-old girl with Poland's Syndrome, introduced lipomodelling as a novel technique for reconstruction of the severe form of the disease. With serial fat injections alone (five sessions over a 2-year period) a breast of natural shape, sensibility, and consistency was created. Relative drawbacks cited by the authors included tedious fat harvesting, the need for multiple sessions, and a partial resorption rate of 30 %. Patient satisfaction, however, was high and longevity of the reconstructive outcome was maintained over the 6-year follow-up period reported. A successful outcome in such a challenging case illustrates the exciting potential of autologous fat injection, a major therapeutic advance in the field of soft tissue reconstruction.

## Conclusion

Poland's Syndrome is a unilateral, congenital disorder of the thorax, breast, and ipsilateral upper extremity. Variability in skeletal and soft tissue deformity is the norm, resulting in a spectrum of severity. Absence of the sternocostal head of the pectoralis major muscle is consistent in all cases and is pathognomonic for the disease.

The goals of surgical correction in Poland's Syndrome are an improvement in chest wall symmetry and, in the female patient, reconstruction of the hypoplastic breast. Creation of an anterior axillary fold and softening of the infraclavicular hollow are the keys to an acceptable result. Underlying skeletal deformity, if present, should be addressed to provide a solid platform for overlying soft tissue reconstruction.

It must be remembered, however, that, with few exceptions, Poland's Syndrome is an aesthetic deformity. The perceived need for reconstruction, therefore, is personal. The patient must decide to what degree he or she is bothered by the deformity, and to what extent he or she is willing

to go to have it corrected. The surgeon, armed with an understanding of the many surgical options available, can then assist the patient in selecting the best reconstructive approach. An individualized approach should be developed, weighing the potential aesthetic gains against the associated morbidity of the various treatment options.

Implant-based breast reconstruction remains a mainstay of treatment for the female patient with Poland's Syndrome. Autologous fat grafting can be used alone or in conjunction with other techniques to help patients achieve an optimal reconstruction.

## References

1. Seyfer A, Fox J. Setting the record straight: the real history of Poland's syndrome. Bull Am Coll Surg. 2012;97(3):27–9.
2. Seyfer AE, Fox JP, Hamilton CG. Poland's syndrome: evaluation and treatment of the chest wall in 63 patients. Plast Reconstr Surg. 2010;126(3):902–11.
3. Poland A. Deficiency of the pectoral muscles. Guys Hosp Rep. 1841;6:191–3.
4. Lallemand LM. Absence de trois cotes simulant un enforcement accidental. Éphémér Méd Montpellier. 1826;1:144–7.
5. Leinveber. Lahmung und Atrophie des linken grossen Brustmuscklels. Med Ztg Berl. 1837;vi:143.
6. Froriep R. Observation of a case of absence of the breast (in German). Notizen Geb Nat Heilkd. 1839;10:9–14.
7. Clarkson P. Poland's syndactyly. Guys Hosp Rep. 1962;111:335–46.
8. Clarkson JH, Harley OJ, Kirkpatrick JJ. Alfred Poland's syndrome: a tidy little controversy. J Plast Reconstr Aesthet Surg. 2006;59:1006–8.
9. Baudinne P, Bovy GL, Wasterain A. A case of Poland's syndrome (in French). Acta Paediatr Belg. 1967;32:407–10.
10. Fokin AA, Robiscek F. Poland's syndrome revisited. Ann Thorac Surg. 2002;74:2218–25.
11. Moir CR, Johnson CH. Poland's syndrome. Semin Pediatr Surg. 2008;17:161–6.
12. Bavnick JNB, Weaver DD. Subclavian artery supply disruption sequence: hypothesis of a vascular etiology for Poland, Klippel-Feil, and Mobius anomalies. Am J Med Genet. 1986;23:903–18.
13. Merlob P, Schonfeld A, Ovadia Y, Reisner SH. Real-time echo-Doppler Duplex Scanner in the evaluation of patients with Poland's sequence. Eur J Obstet Gynecol Reprod Biol. 1989;32:103–8.

14. Bouvet J-P, Leveque D, Bernetieres F, Gros JJ. Vascular origin of Poland syndrome. Eur J Pediatr. 1978;128:17–26.

15. Beer GM, Kompatscher P, Hergan K. Poland's syndrome and vascular malformations. Brit J Plast Surg. 1996;49:482–4.

16. Soltan HC, Holmes LB. Familial occurrence of malformations possibly attributable to vascular abnormalities. J Pediatr. 1986;108:112–4.

17. Sujansky E, Riccardi VM, Matthew AL. The familial occurrence of Poland syndrome. The National Foundation-Birth Defects: Original Article Series1977;XIII:117–21.

18. Fokin AA, Steuerwald NM, Ahrens WA, Allen KE. Anatomical, histologic, and genetic characteristics of congenital chest wall deformities. Semin Thorac Cardiovasc Surg. 2009;21:44–57.

19. Paladini D, D'Armiento MR, Martinelli P. Prenatal ultrasound diagnosis of Poland syndrome. Obstet Gynecol. 2004;104:1156–9.

20. Al-Qattan MM. Classification of hand anomalies in Poland's syndrome. Br J Plast Surg. 2001;54:132–6.

21. Pryor LS, Lehman Jr JA, Workman MC. Disorders of the female breast in the pediatric age group. Plast Reconstr Surg. 2009;124 Suppl 1:50e–60.

22. Ravitch MM. The operative treatment of pectus excavatum. Ann Surg. 1949;129:429–44.

23. Ravitch MM, Handlesman JC. Lesions of the thoracic parietes in infants and children. Deformities and tumors of the chest wall, abnormalities of the diaphragm. Surg Clin North Am. 1952;1397–1424.

24. Ravitch MM. Poland's syndrome. In: Ravitch MM, editor. Congenital deformities of the chest wall and their operative correction. Philadelphia, London, Toronto: WB Saunders; 1977. p. 233–71.

25. Haller Jr JA, Scherer LR, Turner CS, Colombani PM. Evolving management of pectus excavatum based on a single institutional experience of 664 patients. Ann Surg. 1989;209(5):578–82. Discussion 582–3.

26. Haller Jr JA, Colombani PM, Humphries CT, Azizkhan RG, Loughlin GM. Chest wall constriction after too extensive and too early operations for pectus excavatum. Ann Thorac Surg. 1996;61(6):1618–24. Discussion 1625.

27. Fonkalsrud EW. Open repair of pectus excavatum with minimal cartilage resection. Ann Surg. 2004;240(2):231–5.

28. Nuss D, Kelly Jr RE, Croitoru DP, Katz ME. A 10-year review of a minimally invasive technique for the correction of pectus excavatum. J Pediatr Surg. 1998;33(4):545–52.

29. Shamberger RC, Welch KJ, Upton III J. Surgical treatment of thoracic deformity in Poland's syndrome. J Pediatr Surg. 1989;24(8):760–6.

30. Haller Jr JA, Colombani PM, Miller D, Manson P. Early reconstruction of Poland's syndrome using autologous rib grafts combined with a latissimus muscle flap. J Pediatr Surg. 1984;19:423–9.

## Luis Godoy and Gary Raff

## Introduction

There are many variations of sternal anatomy and development. Most of these do not alter chest physiology significantly and as such are not clinically important. Those that do often require surgical treatment early in life. In this chapter, we will review normal sternal development, congenital sternal anomalies and their treatment, and acquired sternal anomalies. Many of the congenital anomalies are often associated with other conditions that result in alterations in the development of other midline structures or thoracic organs.

## Normal Sternal Development

Sternal development begins during the sixth week of gestation. Initially, two sternal bars are seen that fuse at the midline [1, 2]. The fusion

L. Godoy, M.D.
Department of Surgery, University of California,
Davis Medical Center, Sacramento, CA, USA

G. Raff, M.D. (✉)
Department of Surgery, Pediatric Heart Center,
University of California, Davis, 2315 Stockton Blvd.,
Suite 7133, Sacramento, CA, USA
e-mail: gwraff@ucdavis.edu

occurs craniocaudally until it is complete during the tenth week of gestation. After fusion, the osseous segments further develop over the next 20 or so weeks into four or five osseous rests. The superior most osseous rest forms the manubrium while the more inferior osseous rests ultimately fuse during childhood in a caudal to cranial direction. See Fig. 7.1.

During normal growth and development, the primary ossification centers enlarge and fuse to form the adult sternal body while the superior most ossification center forms the manubrium. This process is completed once somatic growth is complete. At various time points during development this process can be disturbed either due to arrest of development or environmental factors that alter maturation.

Failure of fusion or failure in the formation of the sternal bars results in a sternal defect. These defects may occur anywhere along the sternum. Small areas within the sternum where there is a failure of fusion form sternal foramina, if they extend from superior or inferior or if there is complete failure to fuse they form sternal clefts. The superior sternal cleft is thought to be due primarily to lack of development of the manubrium rather than lack of fusion of the sternal bars. Between 30 and 33 weeks gestation the four or five ossification centers can be seen by ultrasound and sternal clefts can be identified at this time [3].

© Springer International Publishing Switzerland 2017
G.W. Raff, S. Hirose (eds.), *Surgery for Chest Wall Deformities*,
DOI 10.1007/978-3-319-43926-6_7

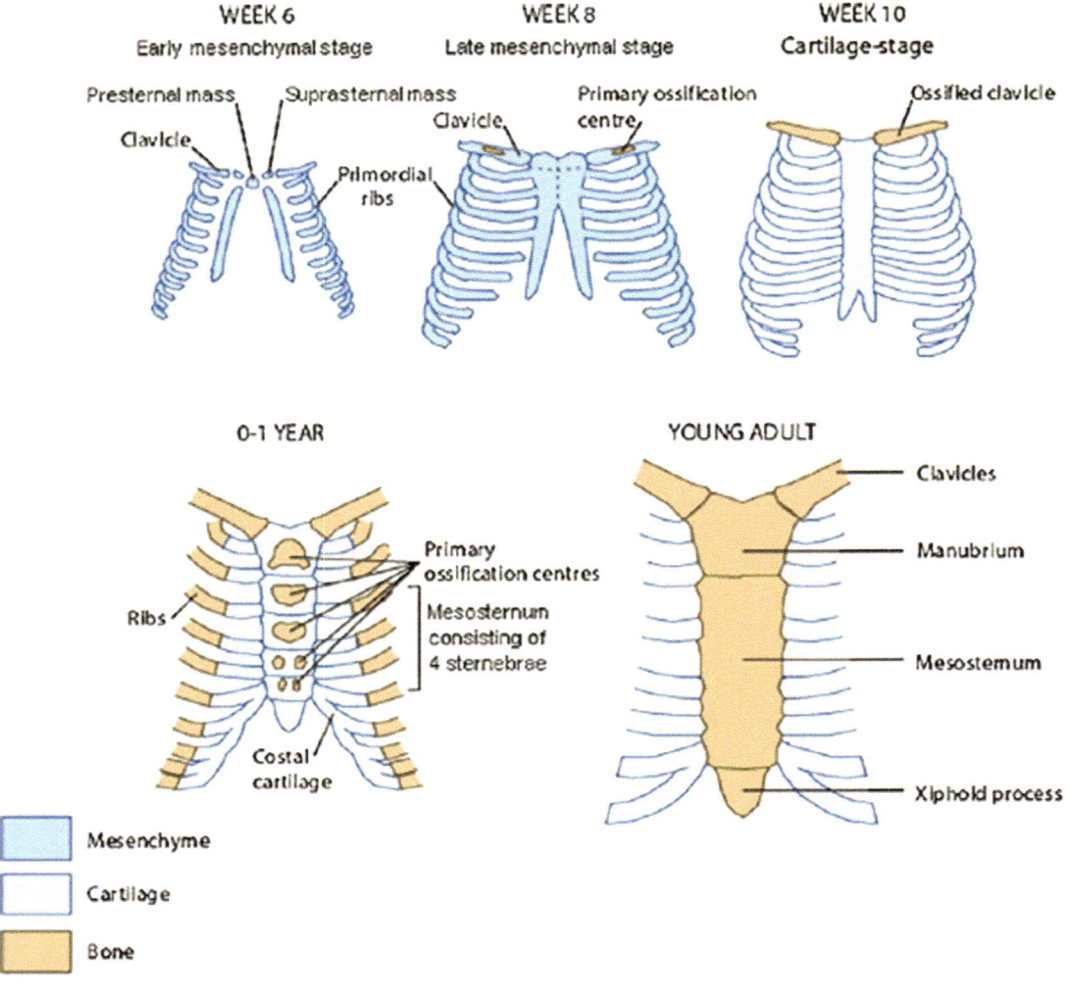

**Fig. 7.1** Human sternal development. Development continues after birth until somatic growth is completed [from van der Merwe, A.E., et al., A review of the embryological development and associated developmental abnormalities of the sternum in the light of a rare palaeopathological case of sternal clefting. Homo, 2013. 64(2): p. 129–41]

## Associated Conditions

Sternal defects, while rare, have a strong association with life-threatening congenital deformities of thoracic and abdominal organs. The presence of a sternal defect should prompt a thorough evaluation of the thoracic cavity, abdomen, and a genetic evaluation. A broad spectrum of deformities have been described involving the sternum, heart, vasculature, and upper abdominal wall. Cardiac anomalies may include ventricular septal defect, double-outlet right ventricle, valvular pathology, and conotruncal anomalies such as Tetralogy of Fallot. Hypoplastic left heart syndrome has been described as well. An association between midline defects and cardiac diseases was made in the 1950's. This was first described by Cantrell in 1958 with findings including: a midline supra-umbilical thoraco-abdominal wall defect, a lower sternal defect, a diaphragmatic pericardial defect, a deficiency of anterior diaphragm and, various intracardiac anomalies [4]. We now refer to this group of defects as Pentalogy of Cantrell. The proposed mechanism is a failure of the lateral mesodermal folds to migrate to the midline, causing the sternal and abdominal defects along with defects in the anterior diaphragm and pericardium. Sternal and abdominal wall defects cause herniation of organs, leading to ectopia cordis and omphalocele. The gene or genes responsible for this have been mapped to the X chromosome (Xq25-Xq26). The syndrome has an estimated incidence of 5.5 per one million live births [5]. Diagnoses of complete pentalogy of Cantrell are extremely rare. Most diagnosed cases are classified as incomplete variants with the subjects meeting three or four out of the five criteria [6]. In addition, some cases describe an association of sternal malformation with other vascular anomalies and vascular dysplasia such as giant ascending aortic aneurysm, aortic coarctation, and coronary ostial abnormalities [7]. It may be that the mesoderm that is important for normal chest wall development also plays a role in development of the conotruncus.

Sternal defects can also be associated with superficial craniofacial vascular lesions. Clinical features associated with this condition include cutaneous craniofacial hemangiomas, sternal cleft, atrophic abdominal raphe extending from the sternal defect to the umbilicus, and associated vascular malformations on internal organs such as the respiratory tract and visceral organs [8]. This spectrum may represent part of the PHACES (Posterior fossa malformations–hemangiomas–arterial anomalies–cardiac defects–eye abnormalities–sternal cleft and supraumbilical raphe) syndrome. Children with sternal malformation and hemangiomas should be carefully evaluated for cardiac, ophthalmologic, and neurologic malformations. The syndrome has an X-linked inheritance pattern and is therefore much more common in females than in males (8:1).

## Diagnosis

The diagnosis of sternal malformation is easily done at birth by physical exam. The most striking finding is one of bulging of the skin overlying a partial sternal cleft or in the case of complete sternal cleft, the precordial pulse. In inferior sternal clefts often associated conditions as mentioned earlier can be seen. Prenatal diagnosis is possible. As previously mentioned, sternal defects are associated with other life-threatening malformations, thus diagnostic investigations have been directed to exclude those associated anomalies. Ultrasonography has been widely used to assess fetal development and has been reported to be of use in early diagnosis. The use of two-dimensional and three-dimensional ultrasonography has been used for early diagnosis and referral to specialized centers [9, 10].

## Sternal Clefts

The exact incidence of sternal malformation is unknown, but it seems to have a 2:1 female predominance [11]. In most cases, infants with sternal cleft are asymptomatic and surgical repair can be performed to provide protective coverage of the underlying heart. The most common of this group of congenital chest wall malformations, this arises from failure of the embryonic fusion of the sternal bars. The defect can be either complete or partial. In a recent review of congenital sternal anomalies, 67 % were superior clefts, 19.5 % complete, 11 % inferior, and 2.5 % were sternal foramen [11]. Sternal clefts are often seen as part of other rare syndromes such as PHACES, Cantrell's pentalogy, sternal malformation/vascular dysplasia, and other midline defects [11]. See Fig. 7.2.

Surgical repair of sternal clefts is indicated to protect the thoracic or abdominal viscera. There have been many different approaches to closure described in the literature [11] and this speaks to the variability in presentation and in anatomy that is seen with these lesions. Repair with autologous tissue and with prosthetic material has been reported with good results although primary closure and repair is preferable if the patient will tolerate this. See Table 7.1.

**Fig. 7.2** Rare associations with sternal cleft [From Torre, M., et al., Phenotypic spectrum and management of sternal cleft: literature review and presentation of a new series. Eur J Cardiothorac Surg, 2012. 41(1): p. 4–9]

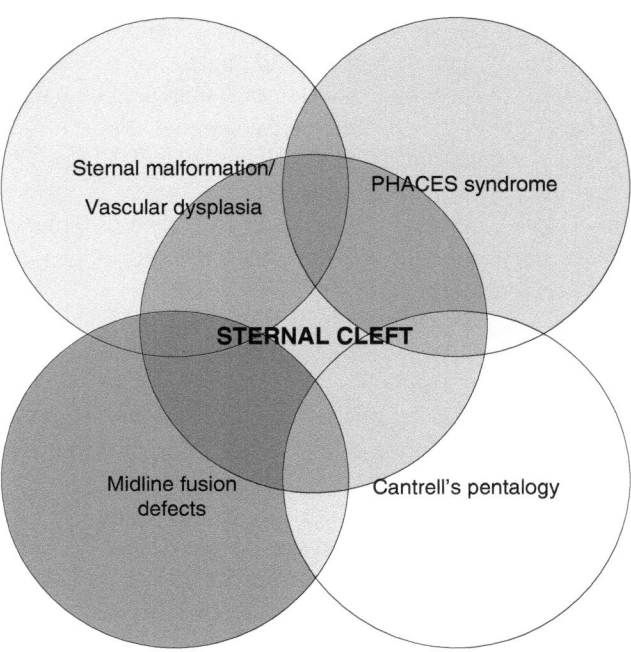

Sternal malformation/
Vascular dysplasia

PHACES syndrome

STERNAL CLEFT

Midline fusion
defects

Cantrell's pentalogy

**Table 7.1** Procedures utilized in repair of sternal clefts adapted from Gaslini [2]

| Surgical procedure | n/70 | % | Gaslini (n/7) | % |
|---|---|---|---|---|
| Primary closure alone | 27 | 38.6 | 4 | 57.14 |
| Primary closure with periosteal flap | 14 | 20.0 | – | – |
| Primary closure with sliding chondrotomies | 10 | 14.3 | – | – |
| Primary closure with cartilage resection | 4 | 5.7 | – | – |
| Bone graft placement | 7 | 10.0 | – | – |
| Prosthetic closure | 5 | 7.1 | 3 | 42.86 |
| Muscle flap | 2 | 2.9 | – | – |
| Two-stage primary closure | 1 | 1.4 | – | – |

## Ectopia Cordis

In this condition, the heart is malpositioned outside of the thoracic cavity and not covered by skin or other somatic structures, known classically as "the naked heart." It was first reported in 1671 by Stensen. The first reported successful repair was at the Children's Hospital of Philadelphia by Koop in 1975. As of 1995 the patient was reported to be alive and well but required multiple reoperations due to the prosthetic material used to reconstruct the anterior chest wall. The apex of the heart is often oriented in the anterior cephalad position and usually has intrinsic anomalies. The sternal defect can be superior, inferior, or total. On rare occasions, the heart may protrude through a defect in the central portion of the sternum. The lack of overlying somatic tissue, along with a hypoplastic thoracic cavity, makes surgical correction very difficult. Isolated survival has been reported in several cases after staged surgeries [12]. See Fig. 7.3. Complicating the management of these patients is the rarity of the lesion combined with the timeliness of surgery that these patients require to survive. Typically these patients do not tolerate repositioning of the heart within the hypoplastic thorax and this is what leads to death. There are numerous different types of ventral wall defects with ectopia cordis [13, 14]. See Table 7.2.

**Fig. 7.3** Total thoracic ectopia cordis [From Alphonso, N., et al., Complete thoracic ectopia cordis. Eur J Cardiothorac Surg, 2003. 23(3): p. 426–8]

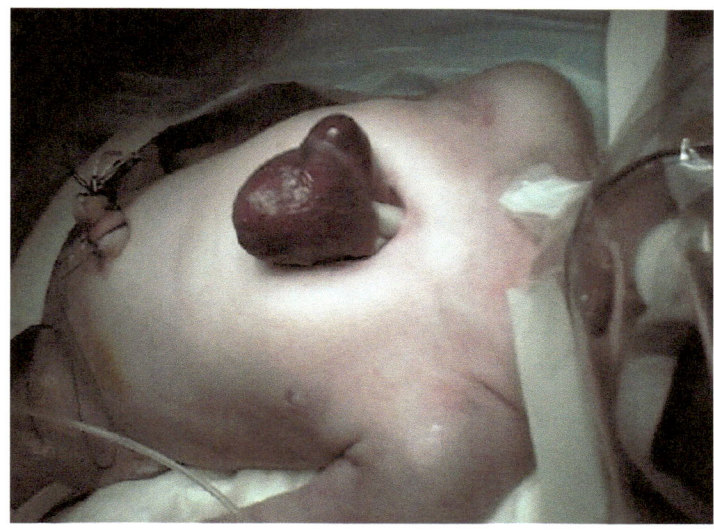

**Table 7.2** Associated anomalies with ectopia cordis [6]

| Sternal defect | No. of cases | Abdominal wall defect | No. of cases | Not reported |
|---|---|---|---|---|
| Completely absent | 10 | Omphalocele | 40 | |
| Xyphoid defect | 10 | Diastasis recti | 15 | |
| Manubrial defect | 3 | Eventration | 8 | |
| Defect of body of sternum | 10 | Umbilical hernia | 3 | |
| Partial defect | 2 | | | |
| One-third lower sternum defect | 24 | | | |
| Two-thirds lower sternum | 11 | | | |
| Bifid sternum | 10 | | | |
| Total | 80 | Total | 66 | 71 |

## Cervical Ectopia Cordis

This is an extremely rare condition in which the heart is displaced cranially, sometimes with the cardiac apex fused with the mouth. These patients usually have severe craniofacial anomalies and often have bands and other anomalies that are not compatible with survival. Prognosis is always poor and there have been no reports of survivors to date.

## Thoraco-Abdominal Ectopia Cordis

The heart is covered by a thin membranous or cutaneous layer that is often pigmented. An inferior sternal cleft is present and the heart can be located within the thorax or be displaced into the abdomen. There are often intrinsic cardiac anomalies present, but there is no cardiac malrotation [15]. This malformation is often found as part of the rare syndrome known as the pentalogy of Cantrell. Cantrell defined this syndrome as having five characteristic findings including omphalocele, anterior diaphragmatic hernia, sternal cleft, ectopia cordis, and an intracardiac defect [4]. Successful repair and long-term survival are much more frequent in thoraco-abdominal ectopia cordis than thoracic ectopia cordis. Ventricular diverticula can also be seen in this condition and are associated with omphalocele and sternal cleft [16]. See Fig. 7.4.

Surgical repair includes reconstruction of the ventral thoracic and abdominal wall as well as diaphragm. Any congenital heart disease present is typically repaired at the time of surgery.

**Fig. 7.4** Ventricular diverticula with
Pentalogy of Cantrell [Nagashima, M.,
T. Higaki, and A. Kurata, Ectopia cordis
with right and left ventricular diverticula.
Heart, 2010. 96(12): p. 973]

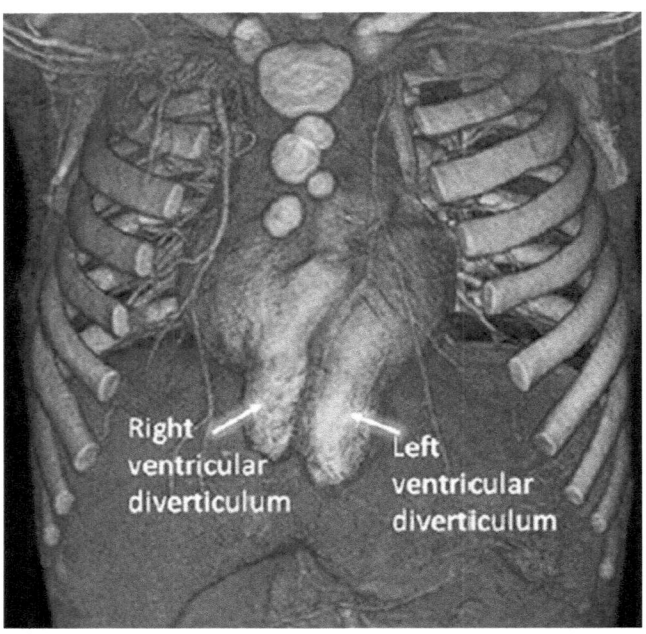

## Treatment of Sternal Deformities

Most cases of sternal cleft are identified at birth.
Conservative treatment and observation is an
acceptable option for asymptomatic patients with
minor defects. For larger defects, surgical
correction is indicated to protect the heart and
major vessels, to improve respiratory dynamics,
and overall development of the thorax.

## Complete Sternal Cleft

Complete sternal clefts should be surgically
repaired whether there are symptoms or not. The
type of operation required to correct a sternal
cleft depends on the age of the patient. Primary
repair should be employed in the neonatal period
because the flexibility of the chest wall is maximal and compression of underlying structures is
minimal. Within the first month of life the defect
can be closed as one would close a median sternotomy in a child of the same age with special
attention being paid to the overlying skin which
can be abnormal and may need to be excised [17].
Ballouhey et al. describe a similar technique.

The surgery is done through a vertical midline
incision. The skin overlying the defect is excised
if it is found to be in direct contact with the pericardium. The sternal bars are dissected and separated from the pericardium in order to preserve
the diaphragmatic nerves. The sternal tables are
freed laterally to the intercostal border. An incision is made on the anterior border of the left sternal bar and on the posterior border of the right
sternal bar and the underlying cartilage exposed
and two perichondrium flaps obtained. The two
sternal bars are then approximated by interrupted
sutures. Close monitoring of the cardiac (heart
rate, systolic blood pressure, and central venous
pressure) and respiratory (tidal volume and pla-
teau pressure) status is then performed for several
minutes to exclude thoracic compartment syndrome before the sutures are tied. Each perichondrial flap is then sutured with the perichondrial
ledge on the opposite sternal bar with absorbable
sutures resulting in a double perichondrium layer.
The subcutaneous tissues and skin are then closed
over the sternum [18]. See Figs. 7.5 and 7.6.

Patients with sternal cleft may present outside
of the neonatal period, late in the childhood or
even in adolescence [19]. Typically after 3
months of age, the chest wall becomes relatively

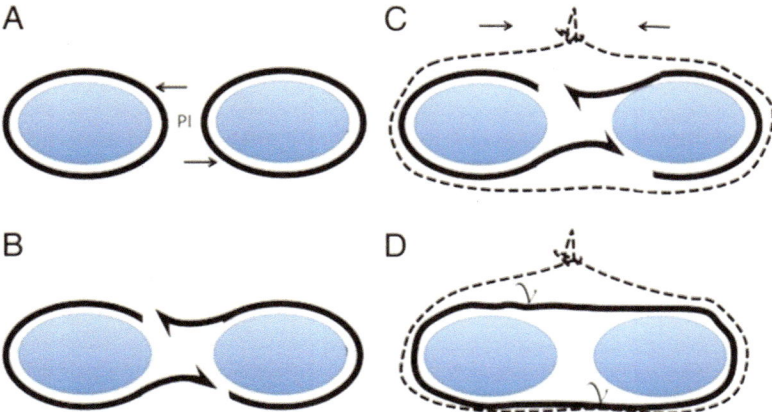

Coronal view of the sternal halves. (A) Asymmetric perichondrium incision (PI), (B) the two elevated flaps are gently elevated, (C) braided non-absorbable interrupted sutures (dotted line) approximate the sternal bars and (D) Each perichondrium flap is sutured to the opposite one

**Fig. 7.5** Creation of perichondral flaps in complete sternal cleft [Ballouhey, Q., et al., Primary repair of sternal cleft with a double osteochondroplasty flap. Interact Cardiovasc Thorac Surg, 2013. 17(6): p. 1036–7]

**Fig. 7.6** Primary repair of complete sternal cleft. (**a**) Operative view after sternal reconstruction. O: place of the osteotomy. *Arrows*: intercostal braided nonabsorbable interrupted sutures. S: superficial perichondrium suture. (**b**) Photograph showing the cosmetic result. The follow-up at 4 months after primary closure of sternal cleft. [Ballouhey, Q., et al., Primary repair of sternal cleft with a double osteochondroplasty flap. Interact Cardiovasc Thorac Surg, 2013. 17(6): p. 1036–7]

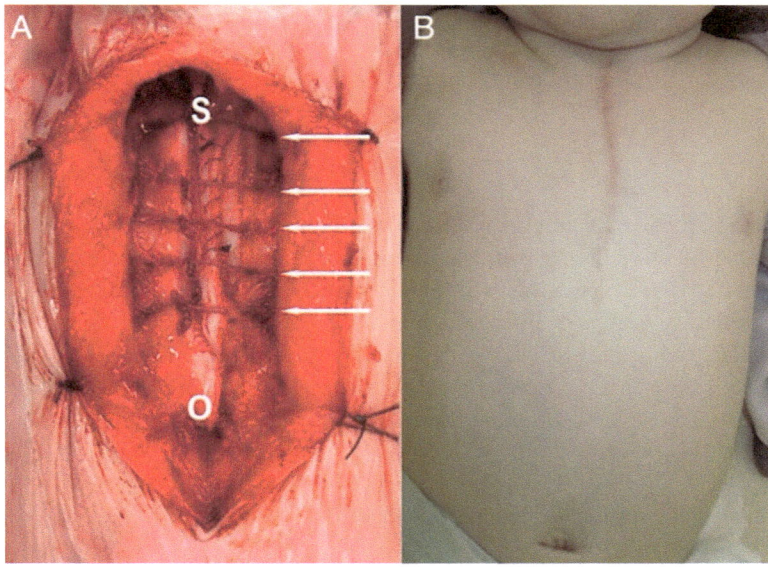

rigid and more complicated techniques may be required [20]. The type of repair is dependent upon the age at presentation, size of the defect, associated conditions, and how well the repair is tolerated physiologically. Techniques that may be required include sliding plasty of the costal cartilages, use of autologous tissue to bridge the gap, or the use of prosthetic material.

## Partial Sternal Cleft

Repair of bifid sternum is best performed through a longitudinal incision extending the length of the defect. Directly beneath the subcutaneous tissues the sternal bars are encountered, with pectoral muscles present lateral to the bars. The endothoracic fascia is mobilized off the sternal bars

**Fig. 7.7** Primary closure technique for sternal clefts [Shamberger, R.C. and K. Welch, Sternal defects. Pediatr Surg Int, 1990(5): p. 156–164]

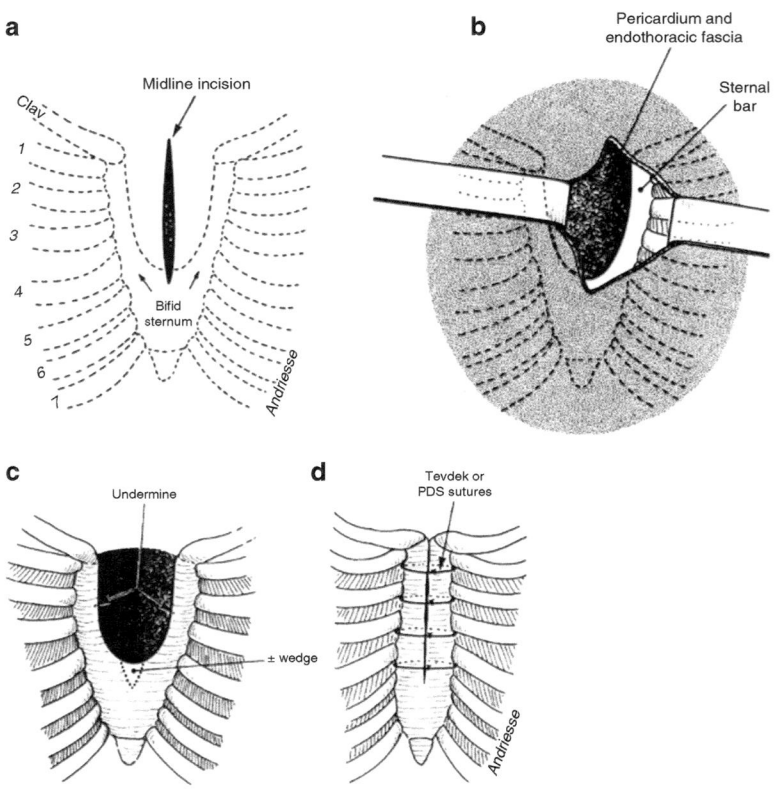

## More Complex Anterior Chest Wall Anomalies

posteriorly with blunt dissection to allow safe placement of the sutures. Approximation of the sternal bars is sometimes facilitated by excising a wedge of cartilage inferiorly which allows for improved apposition of the superior portion of the sternal bars. Closure of the defect is achieved with interrupted suture [21]. See Fig. 7.7.

## More Complex Anterior Chest Wall Anomalies

These include Pentalogy of Cantrell, Ectopia Cordis, Conjoined Twins, and others which are discussed further in other chapters (i.e., pouter pigeon chest, Poland syndrome). These anomalies by definition involve multiple organ systems. Typically the musculoskeletal, cardiac, and pulmonary systems are involved but other systems including the hepatic and gastrointestinal systems can be directly involved as well. These patients

are a technical challenge for the surgeons involved and also are challenging to care for preoperatively and postoperatively. In addition, every case is not quite the same and this often presents unique challenges. As such, we will describe an overall approach to these patients.

Initial therapy should be focused on stabilization and prevention of damage in the event of exposed viscera. A complete evaluation of all organ systems potentially involved must be done and often requires testing such as CT scan and MRI scans, and echocardiogram. A multidisciplinary team approach is mandatory and includes pediatric anesthesia, pediatric surgery, pediatric cardiac surgery, and medical specialists including pediatric critical care and often pediatric cardiology. Once all anomalies have been identified then surgical repair must focus on the following: (1) Establishing either normal cardiac physiology or survivable cardiac physiology, (2) providing normal or survivable pulmonary physiology, (3) providing adequate protection for thoracic and abdominal viscera, and (4) identification of likely postoperative issues so that a proactive approach to prevention or mitigation of these issues can be applied. The following cases will demonstrate this approach.

## Patient Example 1

Newborn with pulsatile mass in the abdominal wall just above the umbilicus. There was an omphalocele noted. No dyspnea and normally saturated. CXR showed dextroposition of the heart and echocardiogram showed a long left ventricular diverticulum extending from the left ventricular apex to the abdomen. CT scan showed an inferior sternal cleft, ventral diaphragmatic hernia, absence of the apex of the pericardium, and the left ventricular diverticulum described earlier. The diagnosis of Pentalogy of Cantrell was made. Anticipated complications for this patient include strangulation of the diverticulum, herniation of abdominal contents into the chest, and hemodynamic instability when closing the cleft over the heart. The surgical plan included the following to mitigate these issues: (1) Resection of the ventricular diverticulum was performed after making a midline sternotomy incision and extending this down to the omphalocele, (2) repair the diaphragm and close the abdominal wall, (3) the sternal cleft was repaired during the course of closing the median sternotomy and repair of the diaphragmatic defect by using a portion of the diaphragm to cover the inferior sternal cleft. Although the heart does not lie in the normal position within the chest after repair, physiologically there is normal heart function [22].

## Patient Example 2

Omphalopagus Conjoined Twins with Shared abdominal wall and liver. Preoperative workup including CT scan, Abdominal Ultrasound, Echocardiogram. A Multispecialty team including Pediatric Surgery, Pediatric Anesthesia, Pediatric Cardiac Surgery, Pediatric Cardiology, and Pediatric Plastic Surgery were involved in workup

and preoperative planning. There was a single shared venous structure running from atrium to atrium between the twins and the pericardium was shared. Anticipated complications included difficulty in closing over the heart due to changes in position that can cause venous inflow occlusion and arterial outflow occlusion as well as frank compression of the heart with closure. The liver could be separated, and the venous connection separated and in one infant the heart was in a fairly normal position although somewhat displaced caudally. After formal separation, the diaphragm was repaired in both infants and in the infant with the caudally displaced heart the closure of the abdominal defect and the pericardium was done with minimal hemodynamic compromise. In the other twin, however, the abdominal defect was larger and the displacement of the heart presented a significant challenge as there were significant beat-to-beat alterations noted with minimal displacement of the ventricle when trying to place it within the chest cavity [see photo]. On further evaluation it became clear that twisting of the pulmonary veins and systemic veins was primarily responsible for this. The venous structures were extensively mobilized to help to mitigate this and the heart was slowly able to be rotated sufficiently to allow closure. Unfortunately, this resulted in a precarious postoperative situation and the patient was very sensitive to position changes and ultimately suffered a fatal cardiac arrest.

## Thoracopagus Twins

Ventral conjoined twins are quite rare and as the case earlier highlights, can be quite challenging to manage. Many cannot be successfully separated due to the complex cardiac anomalies they can have including multichambered hearts. They require an extensive workup and evaluation and the families are counseled extensively on surgical risks and anticipated complications. In ventral conjoined twins there is a very high incidence of congenital heart disease from 10 % in ischiopagus twins to 100 % in thoracopagus twins. The second case above demonstrates very well that the likelihood of success in these patients is dependent upon ability to separate the vital organs and provide adequate coverage of the vital organs in a way that does not alter physiology significantly.

## Acquired Sternal Pathology

With the exception of traumatic injury to the sternum, most acquired sternal lesions are a result of previous surgical intervention. Most common among these is sternal nonunion or sternal infection after median sternotomy. This has been very well studied for decades and the incidence has been fairly static despite improved understanding of the factors that contribute to this. Interruption of the blood supply to the sternum after the Ravitch procedure has resulted in poor growth of the sternum and even thoracic dystrophy. In the current era, it is unusual to see this complication of the Ravitch procedure since we no longer perform this procedure in small children, but rather reserve it for adolescents who have had the majority of their thorax growth already completed. Sternal tumors can also be acquired but as chest wall tumors are covered in another chapter we will not revisit this topic here.

## Sternal Fractures

Traumatic injury to the sternum and chest wall can occur from any blunt force to the anterior chest such as motor vehicle accident, gunshot wounds, or even CPR [23, 24]. The major tenants for treatment are similar to that in other orthopedic trauma including rigid fixation and stabilization when there is significant dislocation or sternal instability. One of the unique issues to consider with sternal injury is the treatment of pain. Inadequate pain control has been shown to result in significant pulmonary morbidity [25]. Therefore, most treatment algorithms include regional blocks for pain control, and often early rigid fixation to help reduce pain and allow earlier return to ambulation and mobility.

Sternal fixation can be done using a variety of techniques including suture or wire, and plating systems that can be permanent or absorbable. Each of these techniques has their merits and detractors. There is no best technique to use in every patient so surgeons must be familiar with a variety of techniques in order to best treat their patients. In our center, we typically will utilize standard sternal wires for fractures or cuts that are longitudinal, similar to how a midline sternotomy is closed. If we are concerned about the potential for wires to pull through the sternum we will consider surgical "zip ties" or nonabsorbable plates and screws. For other fractures we would typically utilize plates and screws. We have utilized both absorbable and nonabsorbable plates and screws. We have had numerous patients present to our clinic with chest wall pain after repair of sternal fracture and on workup discovered fractured rib fixation hardware that was utilized to provide rigid fixation for a sternal fracture, therefore we do not advise utilizing rib fixation hardware to provide sternal stabilization or if this hardware is used, then recommend removing the hardware once the sternum has healed.

## Sternal Infections

Although the majority of sternal infections are in the setting of previous median sternotomy, there are many reports of sternal osteomyelitis in patients who never had a median sternotomy [26]. The diagnosis of sternal infection can be made clinically if there are typical symptoms including fever, swelling, erythema, warmth, etc. In patients after median sternotomy, identification of sternal instability (either the patient telling you they feel a click or in demonstrating a click with deep inspiration and cough) is common in patients with sternal infection. This can be confirmed with CT or MRI (or in some cases bone scan) and the offending organism isolated so that proper therapy can be provided. After previous intervention the majority of organisms are Staphlococcal and E. coli and Klebsiella tend to be less common and tend to occur in patients with other infectious complications such as pneumonia, urinary tract infections, and other nosocomial infections. Polymicrobial infections are more common in diabetic patients.

The treatment of sternal infections is predicated upon first identifying the organism(s) responsible. In primary infection, no debridement may be necessary. In typical infection after sternotomy, the area is debrided to viable tissue and then a plan for closure is decided upon. There have been many different strategies developed to accomplish this and no consensus or randomized prospective studies to help guide choice of procedure or protocol can be strongly recommended [27–34]. Factors that have resulted in the greatest success include initial wound treatment with a vacuum system or irrigation system to allow for gross eradication of infection, adequate debridement, closure of the sternum or replacement of the sternum with viable tissue (muscle flaps or omentum), and then adequate soft tissue coverage over drains. The morbidity, mortality, and cost of these infections are significant.

## Summary

Sternal cleft and anomalies are rare. Minor anomalies that do not alter physiology can be treated expectantly. More significant anomalies that leave the thoracic viscera exposed are addressed surgically. Often there are associated conditions that must also be addressed.

## References

1. Mekonen HK, et al. Development of the ventral body wall in the human embryo. J Anat. 2015;227(5): 673–85.
2. van der Merwe AE, et al. A review of the embryological development and associated developmental abnormalities of the sternum in the light of a rare palaeopathological case of sternal clefting. Homo. 2013;64(2):129–41.
3. Pasoglou V, et al. Sternal cleft: prenatal multimodality imaging. Pediatr Radiol. 2012;42(8):1014–6.
4. Cantrell JR, Haller JA, Ravitch MM. A syndrome of congenital defects involving the abdominal wall, sternum, diaphragm, pericardium, and heart. Surg Gynecol Obstet. 1958;107(5):602–14.
5. Carmi R, Boughman JA. Pentalogy of Cantrell and associated midline anomalies: a possible ventral midline developmental field. Am J Med Genet. 1992;42(1):90–5.
6. Toyama WM. Combined congenital defects of the anterior abdominal wall, sternum, diaphragm, pericar-

dium, and heart: a case report and review of the syndrome. Pediatrics. 1972;50(5):778–92.
7. Padalino MA, et al. Giant congenital aortic aneurysm with cleft sternum in a neonate: pathological and surgical considerations for optimal management. Cardiovasc Pathol. 2010;19(3):183–6.
8. Hersh JH, et al. Sternal malformation/vascular dysplasia association. Am J Med Genet. 1985;21(1): 177–86, 201–2.
9. Yang TY, et al. Prenatal diagnosis of pentalogy of Cantrell using three-dimensional ultrasound. Taiwan J Obstet Gynecol. 2013;52(1):131–2.
10. Izquierdo MT, Bahamonde A, Domene J. Prenatal diagnosis of a complete cleft sternum with 3-dimensional sonography. J Ultrasound Med. 2009;28(3):379–83.
11. Torre M, et al. Phenotypic spectrum and management of sternal cleft: literature review and presentation of a new series. Eur J Cardiothorac Surg. 2012;41(1):4–9.
12. Dobell AR, Williams HB, Long RW. Staged repair of ectopia cordis. J Pediatr Surg. 1982;17(4):353–8.
13. Leca F, et al. Extrathoracic heart (ectopia cordis). Report of two cases and review of the literature. Int J Cardiol. 1989;22(2):221–8.
14. Alphonso N, Venugopal PS, Anderson D. Complete thoracic ectopia cordis. Eur J Cardiothorac Surg. 2003;23:426–8.
15. Major JW. Thoracoabdominal ectopia cordis; report of a case successfully treated by surgery. J Thorac Surg. 1953;26(3):309–17.
16. Nagashima M, Higaki T, Kurata A. Ectopia cordis with right and left ventricular diverticula. Heart. 2010;96(12):973.
17. Firmin RK, Fragomeni LS, Lennox SC. Complete cleft sternum. Thorax. 1980;35(4):303–6.
18. Ballouhey Q, et al. Primary repair of sternal cleft with a double osteochondroplasty flap. Interact Cardiovasc Thorac Surg. 2013;17(6):1036–7.
19. Yavuzer S, Kara M. Primary repair of a sternal cleft in an infant with autogenous tissues. Interact Cardiovasc Thorac Surg. 2003;2(4):541–3.
20. Fokin AA. Cleft sternum and sternal foramen. Chest Surg Clin N Am. 2000;10(2):261–76.
21. Shamberger RC, Welch K. Sternal defects. Pediatr Surg Int. 1990;5:156–64.
22. Di Bernardo S, Sekarski N, Meijboom E. Left ventricular diverticulum in a neonate with Cantrell syndrome. Heart. 2004;90(11):1320.
23. Olds K, Byard RW, Langlois NE. Injuries associated with resuscitation — an overview. J Forensic Leg Med. 2015;33:39–43.
24. Kralj E, et al. Frequency and number of resuscitation related rib and sternum fractures are higher than generally considered. Resuscitation. 2015;93:136–41.
25. Thomas KP, et al. Ultrasound-guided parasternal block allows optimal pain relief and ventilation improvement after a sternal fracture. Pain Ther. 2016;5(1):115–22.
26. Young Ann J, et al. Sternal osteomyelitis with a mediastinal abscess caused by Gemella morbillorum fol-

lowing blunt force trauma. Intern Med. 2013;52(4): 511–4.

27. Vaziri M, Jesmi F, Pishgahroudsari M. Omentoplasty in deep sternal wound infection. Surg Infect (Larchmt). 2015;16(1):72–6.

28. Eburdery H, et al. Management of large sternal wound infections with the superior epigastric artery perforator flap. Ann Thorac Surg. 2016;101(1):375–7.

29. Caballero MJ, et al. Aspergillus mediastinitis after cardiac surgery. Int J Infect Dis. 2016;44:16–9.

30. Seng P, et al. Osteomyelitis of sternum and rib after breast prosthesis implantation: a rare or underestimated infection? IDCases. 2015;2(1):31–3.

31. Marano AA, Feintisch AM, Granick MS. Omental flap for thoracic aortic graft infection. Eplasty. 2015;15:ic41.

32. Listewnik MJ, et al. The use of vacuum-assisted closure in purulent complications and difficult-to-heal wounds in cardiac surgery. Adv Clin Exp Med. 2015;24(4):643–50.

33. Lee JC, Raman J, Song DH. Primary sternal closure with titanium plate fixation: plastic surgery effecting a paradigm shift. Plast Reconstr Surg. 2010;125(6): 1720–4.

34. Lee JH, et al. Primary sternal osteomyelitis caused by actinomyces israelii. Korean J Thorac Cardiovasc Surg. 2015;48(1):86–9.

# Chest Wall Tumors

Sabrina A. Oldfield and Elizabeth A. David

## Introduction

The musculoskeletal structure of the chest wall serves to protect the thoracic and mediastinal viscera, while providing integrity for respiration. The complex relationship of all anatomic components contributes to its function but also makes it susceptible to a wide variety of pathology. Thus, tumors of the chest wall represent a diagnostic and therapeutic challenge. Chest wall masses have a broad differential diagnosis including local extension of intrathoracic lesions, presentations of systemic diseases or inflammatory processes, metastasis, and less frequently, primary tumors of the chest wall, which can be benign or malignant. More than 50 % are malignant and are most commonly a result of direct invasion or metastasis from adjacent thoracic tumors [1]. Overall, primary chest wall tumors make up less than 5 % of thoracic malig-

S.A. Oldfield, M.D.
Section of General Thoracic Surgery, Department of Surgery, UC Davis Medical Center, Sacramento, CA, USA

E.A. David, M.D., F.A.C.S. (✉)
Section of General Thoracic Surgery, Department of Surgery, UC Davis Medical Center, Sacramento, CA, USA

Heart Lung Vascular Center, David Grant Medical Center, Travis AFB, Sacramento, CA, USA
e-mail: eadavid@ucdavis.edu

nancies and vary widely in pathology, as they arise from all anatomic structures comprising the chest wall [2, 3]. This chapter reviews the pathology, options for diagnosis, and standard treatment of the various lesions arising from the chest wall.

## Evaluation

### Signs and Symptoms/Clinical Presentation

Chest wall tumors, with their diverse etiology, also have varying clinical presentations. Workup should always begin with a thorough history and physical. They can be symptomatic or asymptomatic, with >20 % being found incidentally on chest radiograph [4]. Pain is the most common symptom for both benign and malignant lesions and it is usually a sign of bony invasion. Extrathoracic tumors are more likely to present as a palpable, enlarging mass, which is a common presentation, along with pain. There is a wide variation of age at presentation. Older patients tend to have larger, more aggressive tumors when compared to their younger counterparts, who are more likely to have smaller benign tumors [4]. Though tumors can present at any age, they are more likely to be malignant at the extremes of age [3]. There are no specific signs or symptoms that distinguish between benign and malignant lesions, which add to the challenge of diagnosis [3]. Symptoms can indicate the location of the lesion, for instance, paresthesia and weakness may be present with involvement of neurologic structures.

## Diagnosis

To perform an operation with the best possible outcome for the patient, correct diagnosis, preoperative staging, and surgical planning are essential. Given the wide variation in histology of origin, it is frequently necessary to use imaging appearance, location, and clinical information to make a diagnosis rather than imaging alone [5].

## Imaging Modalities

*Chest Radiograph*: Radiographic diagnosis alone can be challenging. As mentioned previously, >20 % of chest wall tumors are found incidentally on chest x-ray [5]. If this is not the case, chest radiograph is often the first imaging modality obtained [6]. The chest radiograph can not only show location and size, it can detect calcification, ossification, or bone destruction, but is otherwise limited in detail. Therefore, additional workup is always indicated, with CT and MRI being the most useful diagnostic modalities (Fig. 8.1).

*Computed Tomography (CT)*: If contrast is used, CT scan can provide information about the vascularity of a tumor, location, and composition of a chest wall mass, as well as appraisal of the extent of tumor invasion and involved structures. It is also better at predicting cortical bone involvement. Cartilaginous matrix calcifications are better defined with CT than with MRI which is very useful for preoperative planning [6]. It can also be useful in confirming histologic diagnosis by obtaining a CT-guided biopsy of a lesion. The approach for biopsy should be chosen together with the surgeon, with consideration given for preoperative planning (Fig. 8.2).

*Magnetic Resonance Imaging (MRI)*: Accurate tissue characterization can be obtained with MRI due to its superior tissue-resolving features and multiplanar image acquisition, which makes it an important assessment tool [5, 7].·It is the most accurate study for spinal involvement, characterizing soft tissue involvement, and further delineating between vascular, soft tissue, and nerve involvement [3, 6, 8] (Fig. 8.3).

*Positron Emission Tomography (PET)*: The clinical significance of standard uptake value (SUV) may be useful but has not been formally established as a diagnostic tool in the evaluation of chest wall lesions [9, 10]. There is some data suggesting that PET may be more accurate for determining the extent of large tumors, especially those >5.5 cm [10, 11]. Though, it is not routinely

**Fig. 8.1** Chest radiograph of large left chest wall tumor found to be poorly differentiated carcinoma with extensive necrosis

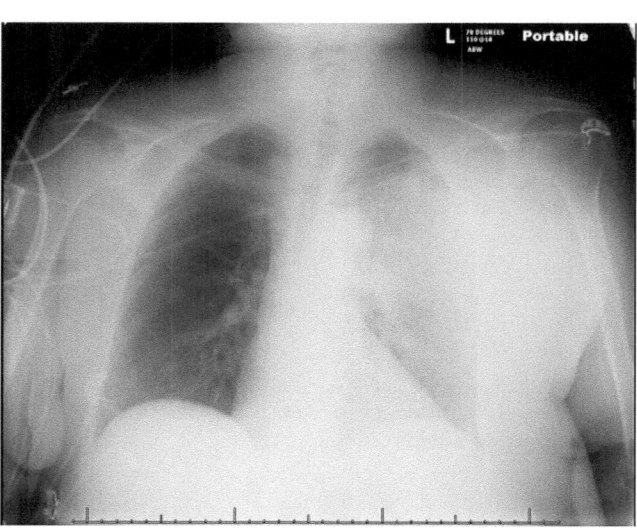

**Fig. 8.2**  Axial CT scan of chest wall sarcoma demonstrating osseous destruction of right anterior third rib

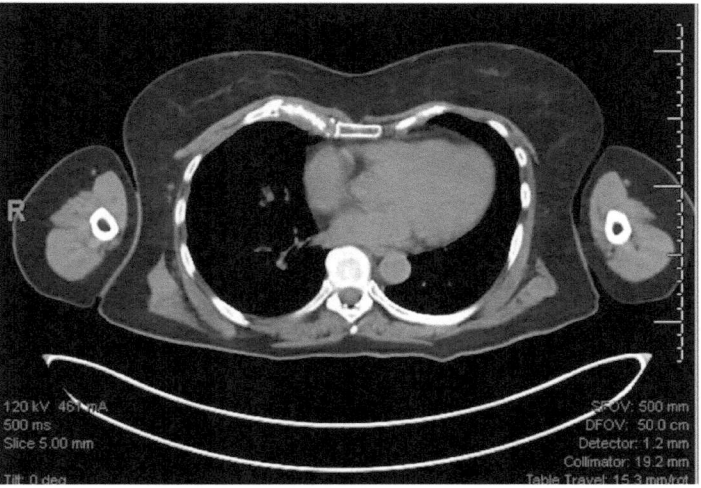

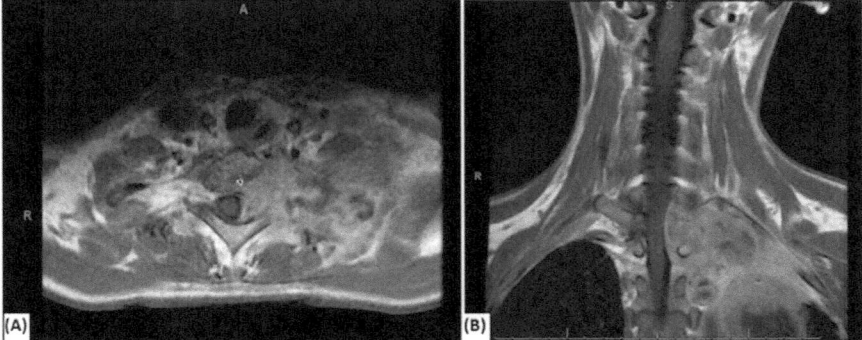

**Fig. 8.3**  MRI scan of left chest tumor in a patient with Hodgkin's Lymphoma invading the thoracic spine causing cord displacement and rib destruction (**a**) axial view and (**b**) coronal view

discussed as a common imaging modality in the evaluation of chest wall tumors, there seems to be increasing frequency of its mention in the literature. In a small recent study by Petermann et al., PET imaging was found to be superior to CT for defining the extent of chest wall tumors, giving hope that it will be found to be of significant diagnostic value in larger prospective studies, which have yet to be conducted [11]. In the case of malignant disease, it may be useful for defining patients with limited disease versus disseminated disease (Fig. 8.4).

*Ultrasound* (*US*): There has recently been documented use of ultrasound for more clearly defining tumor margins [6, 10, 12]. Ultrasound may accurately predict the degree of tumor inva-sion or extension, which could help with preoperative planning to ensure negative surgical margins [10]. Caroli et al. describe the absence of lung sliding on ultrasound as being accurately predictive for lung invasion from a chest wall tumor in 8/8 patients where other imaging modalities were inconclusive [12].

## Biopsy

In the majority of cases, radiographic features alone are insufficient to make a complete diagnosis; therefore, histologic evaluation is required. Suitable modalities to obtain tissue diagnosis include fine-needle aspiration, incisional biopsy,

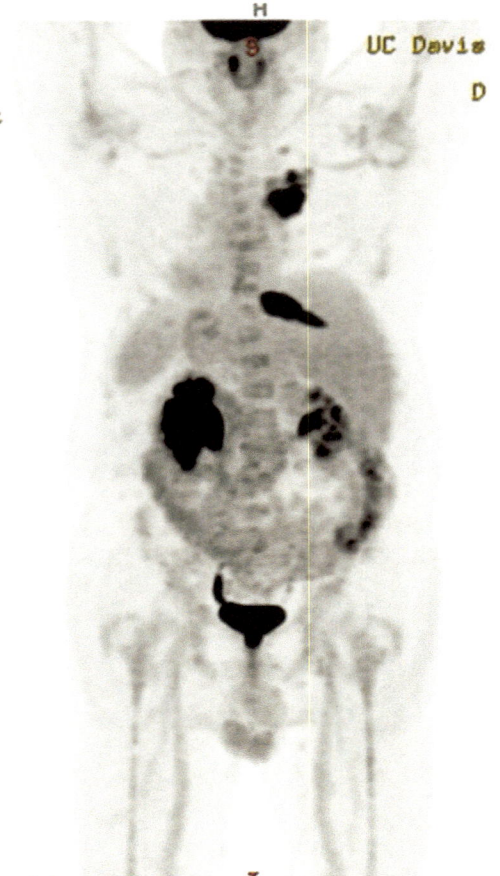

**Fig. 8.4** Maximum Intensity Projection image from PET/CT demonstrating isolated metastasis to the right tenth rib from NSCLC

or excisional biopsy [9]. The approach to obtaining a biopsy is guided by the size and location of the lesion, extent of resection, complexity of any associated need for reconstruction, and if there are any associated comorbidities. Typically, lesions less than 2–5 cm undergo excisional biopsy depending on the suspected pathology and the surgical center [2, 3, 10]. An absolute diagnosis prior to resection is usually of value for lesions greater than 5 cm, given the increased likelihood of extensive dissection and complex reconstruction. Therefore, lesions greater than 2–5 cm may undergo needle aspiration or incisional biopsy for confirmation of diagnosis, allowing for better operative planning [2, 3, 10]. Core needle biopsy may determine if it is a benign or malignant pro-

cess but may not obtain sufficient sampling for further histologic analysis or genetic testing.

It is essential that the entire treatment plan be considered before any biopsy to ensure correct placement of the biopsy location. The lesion is often approached directly in order to avoid contamination of surrounding structures. If a malignant diagnosis is obtained, definitive excision is required, which necessitates total excision of the biopsy tract. It is preferable, for the earlier reasons, that the biopsy be performed at the treating/ surgical center rather than at the referring center, or in coordination with the operating surgeon.

## Preoperative Evaluation

Once the diagnosis has been made, and the primary excision is determined, it is important to complete a thorough history and physical with careful consideration of any past surgical history or treatment which may affect approaches for resection or reconstruction. Immunosuppression, history of radiation or planned radiation, and previous chest procedures should all be considered. Additionally, full medical assessment should be obtained, including a cardiac and pulmonary function evaluation in cases where there is concern for simultaneous pulmonary resection. As mentioned earlier, complete radiographic analysis is essential to operative planning and may delineate the need for preoperative consultation with neurosurgical or reconstructive specialists. Patients with extensive or complicated lesions are best served with a multidisciplinary approach, which may include cardiothoracic surgery, spine surgery, plastic surgery, radiation oncology, and/ or medical oncology [10, 13].

## Pathology

### Benign

Benign chest wall tumors are less common than malignant lesions and arise from nerve, blood vessel, osseous, cartilaginous, or fatty tissue [5]. It is crucial that malignant diagnoses are definitively ruled out with radiographic and histologic analysis for any of these lesions.

## Skeletal Lesions

Benign chest wall tumors of bony origin are less common than malignant bony lesions. However, one should always assume a malignant condition until proven otherwise.

### Osteochondroma

Osteocondroma is the most common type of benign bone tumor and is typically found in the femur, humerus, and tibia [14]. In the chest, osteochondromas are most common in the rib or scapula, where they are commonly found at the costochondral junction, and they develop from abnormal growth of normal tissue [5, 10]. Osteochondromas make up 50 % of benign rib tumors [2]. These masses frequently cause pain as they progress with growth of bony exostoses [14]. Peak incidence is in the second decade of life [15]. It is one of the few chest wall tumors where a definitive diagnosis can be made on CT or MRI based on the appearance of the cortex and medullary space blending into the underlying bone [5], and punctate or flocculent calcifications with mineralized hyaline cartilage cap [3]. Surgical treatment is resection and provides complete pathologic evaluation, symptomatic relief, and minimizes the risk of malignant transformation [16]. Cartilage caps greater than 2 cm in adults and greater than 3 cm in children are suspicious for malignant degeneration [3, 10].

### Chondromas (Enchondromas)

Chondromas are also typically found at the sternocostal junction arising from cartilaginous tissue [2, 10]. They are relatively common, making up 15–20 % of benign chest wall lesions. Chondromas are usually painless, slow growing, osteolytic lesions, and present between 20 and 30 years of age. The distinction between chondroma and low-grade chondrosarcoma is difficult. Therefore, all chondromas are treated as malignant lesions, and wide excision is recommended [4]. Appropriate wide excision for a malignant lesion is commonly accepted as full thickness resection with 4-cm margins and en bloc removal of one rib above and below the lesion as well as intercostal muscles, pleura, and wide clear margin of adjacent tissue [17, 18].

### Fibrous Dysplasia

Fibrous dysplasia typically appears in the lateral or posterior tract of the ribs and is the third most frequent benign chest wall lesion [2]. Normal bone is replaced with fibrous tissue forming a slow-growing mass, which can cause pathologic fractures and result in pain; otherwise, presentation may be as an asymptomatic mass in the posterior aspect of a rib. Fibrous dysplasia appears as a lytic lesion on chest radiograph with a soap bubble or ground-glass appearance that is diagnostic. Only one bone is involved in 70–80 % of the cases [5], most commonly the second rib [10]. In 25 % of cases it affects more than one bone [15]. When this occurs, it may also be associated with cafe-au-lait spots and endocrine abnormalities with the constellation of abnormalities known as McCune–Albright syndrome [3, 15]. It typically occurs in the second and third decade of life with no disparity in gender ratio [3]. Treatment is wide local excision for relief of symptoms and confirmation of diagnosis [4]. Conversely, some sources believe that excision is not necessary if the lesion remains asymptomatic, as imaging is often diagnostic [10].

### Eosinophilic Granuloma/Langerhans Cell Histiocytosis

Eosinophilic granuloma, or Langerhans cell histiocytosis, is a less common tumor that can arise in the anterior chest wall [4]. This results from idiopathic proliferation of histiocytes, considered to be of bone marrow origin. These masses tend to present with chest pain, fevers, and an isolated tender mass that has a typical lytic appearance on radiograph and chest CT [19]. Eosinophilic granuloma is a diffuse infiltrative inflammatory process that can affect many organs and can also manifest with an associated leukocytosis. In the chest wall, it can cause destruction of bone cortex and new subperiosteal bone formation that can mimic osteomyelitis or malignancy [4]. Treatment in the literature varies ranging from nonsurgical approaches such as steroids, chemotherapy, and low dose radiotherapy without surgical excision [3] to wide local excision performed both for diagnosis and symptomatic relief [19, 20]. Most forms are treated nonsurgically, but if the lesion is isolated, then resection and curettage are reported to have good results [10]. This lesion requires a histologic diagnosis, with identification of birbeck granules on electron microscopy [3]. If a procedure is necessary for diagnostic purposes, then it often makes sense to pursue excisional biopsy at the time.

## Aneurysmal Bone Cyst

Aneurysmal bone cysts are a rare, benign, locally aggressive entity consisting of an expanding osteolytic lesion with blood-filled cystic spaces. Their etiology is not clear, as they are often associated with abnormal bone or are found in the setting of another underlying bone tumor [10]. They are usually found on the posterior chest wall and 75 % present before the age of 20 [3]. If there is soft tissue extension, then it may be difficult to differentiate from sarcomas. Complete excision is recommended, with cure rates of 70–90 % [10]. Radiation is sometimes used for local control in the setting of aggressive or recurrent tumors [10]. These lesions are not known to metastasize.

## Osteoid Osteomas

Osteoid Osteomas are small, tumors of osteoblastic origin that rarely occur as primary chest wall tumors [15]. They often present in the first and second decades with nocturnal pain, which is improved by NSAIDs [3, 10]. The most common location for presentation is the posterior spine and ribs and can also be associated with scoliosis. Radiographically, they have a small radiolucent lesion with thick sclerotic margin of reactive bone and surrounding soft tissue edema. Their characteristic appearance on bone scan is known as the double density sign [15]. Treatment generally involves radiofrequency ablation.

## Osteoblastoma

Osteoblastoma is a rare osteoblastic tumor thought to be on the continuum of osteoid osteomas [3,

10]. These tumors also primarily affect the posterior ribs. On radiologic evaluation they appear as well-defined expanding osteolytic lesion, but with a sharp sclerotic rim and lack of a central nidus. They can be locally aggressive with potential for recurrence, and thus wide local excision is the preferred treatment [15].

## Giant Cell Tumor

Giant cell tumors are more common and occur most frequently between the second and fourth decades [10], with men having a higher occurrence than women [3]. They are considered locally aggressive with 30–50 % recurrence rates and rare reports of metastasis [3]. Secondary to their locally aggressive nature, wide local excision is recommended [10]. They are osteolytic lesions with cortical thinning and often are associated with a soft tissue mass (Table 8.1).

## Soft Tissue Tumors

Soft tissue tumors that affect the chest wall have a similar variability in pathology of that of the bone-based lesions. Cutaneous nevi, lipomas, hemangiomas, lymphangiomas, and neurogenic tumors are some of the benign lesions that can be found in the soft tissue of the chest wall. They are treated with wide local excision to negative margins to avoid local tissue recurrence. Soft tissue tumors have some additional challenges to preoperative diagnosis. Intercostal hernias have been reported to be confused with benign soft tissue lesions, mandating appropriate radiographic confirmation of clinical suspicion based on history and physical exam [21]. Radiographic evaluation may not always definitively address malignancy but will assist in operative planning.

## Lipomas

Lipomas usually present as well-circumscribed adipose masses but are often deeper and larger on the chest than on other sites of the body [3]. They are more prevalent in the obese and older patients, with incidence highest at approximately ages 50–70 [3]. As with many chest wall tumor presentations, they can sometimes be challenging to

**Table 8.1**  Benign bony lesions

| Tumor | Origin | Presentation | Imaging characteristics | Treatment |
|---|---|---|---|---|
| Osteochondroma | Cartilage | Rib, scapula, 50 % of benign rib tumors. Peak incidence in second decade | Cortex and medullary space blends w/ underlying bone, punctate or flocculent calcifications w/ mineralized hyaline cap (>2 cm cap in adults or >3 cm in children = ↑ risk of malignant transformation) | Resection |
| Chondroma (enchondromas) | Cartilage | Usually painless lesion at 20–30 year of age, most commonly found in anterior ribs | Osteolytic, lobulated appearance with distinct boarders | Wide local excision— distinction from low-grade malignant chondrosarcoma is difficult |
| Fibrous dysplasia | Fibrous tissue | Lateral or posterior rib. Slow growing. Often w/ pathologic fracture @ 20–30 yo | Lytic lesion. Soap bubble or ground glass appearance = diagnostic | Wide local excision for symptoms and definitive diagnosis vs. no intervention if diagnosis confirmed and remains asymptomatic |
| Eosinophilic granuloma (langerhans histiocytosis) | Bone marrow | Anterior chest wall, ribs, sternum. Rare. | Focal lytic radiolucent lesions with biopsy necessary for diagnosis (birbeck granules on histology) | Most forms treated nonsurgically. If the lesion is isolated, then resection and curettage are reported to have good results |
| | | May have pain, fever, leukocytosis | | |
| Giant cell tumor | Osteoclast | 20–40 yo with ♂>♀ | Osteolytic lesions with cortical thinning, often with soft tissue mass | Wide local excision recommended secondary to locally aggressive nature and rare ability to metastasize |
| | | 30–50 % risk of recurrence | Vascular sinuses w/ giant cells and spindle cells | |
| Aneurysmal bone cyst | Unclear | Posterior chest wall, <20 yo, rare, locally aggressive. can coexist with other lesions | Cystic, expanding osteolytic lesions. Free fluid w/ multiseptated hemorrhagic cysts which are not pathognomonic | With complete excision, cure rates 70–90 %. Radiation may be used for aggressive disease or recurrent tumors |
| Osteoid osteoma | Osteoblast | Nocturnal rib pain that responds to NSAIDs and Tylenol, first–second decade of life. Often posterior, may be associated with scoliosis | Small radiolucent lesion with thick sclerotic margin of reactive bone with soft tissue edema. Characteristic appearance on bone scan = double density sign | Radiofrequency ablation? |
| Osteoblastoma | Osteoblast | Posterior/ posterio-lateral rib mass or pain | Well-defined osteolytic lesion with sharp sclerotic rim and lack of a central nidus | Can be locally aggressive and recurs, wide local excision is recommended |

evaluate with radiographic modalities, and are often difficult to differentiate from low-grade liposarcomas [3]. There have been case reports of soft tissue lesions with preoperative imaging suggestive of intrathoracic or chest wall invasion, which were subsequently found to be giant benign lipomas on excision [22, 23]. Chest wall lipomas should be excised for symptomatic relief and complete diagnostic evaluation secondary to the risk of malignant transformation.

## Lymphangiomas

Lymphangiomas of the chest wall can be cystic or cavernous in nature and are a result of a developmental malformation. They can be located within the mediastinum or the chest wall itself. Preoperative CT imaging is essential to assess the extent of the lesion, as several reports of giant lesions exist in the literature [24, 25]. Complete surgical excision is required for excellent prognosis and avoidance of long-term lymphatic fistula formation. Nonoperative therapy with radiation or sclerosing agents remains controversial for lymphangiomas of the chest wall, with surgery as the standard of care [2].

## Hemangiomas

Hemangiomas arise from blood vessels and can be found within the chest wall or protruding through the chest wall from the thoracic cavities or mediastinum and arise from blood vessels. Often seen as heterogeneous soft tissue masses with fatty, fibrous, and vascular elements on CT scan [3]. Ultrasound may be a useful modality to evaluate flow within the lesion [3]. MRI is used to distinguish benign from malignant lesions based on phleboliths, fat component, and high intensity and fat suppression on T2 imaging technique, but surgical biopsy is required for definitive diagnosis [26]. Hemangiomas of the chest wall can be intramuscular, intercostal, or cavernous. They tend to occur in patients less than 30 years of age and present as painful masses. Treatment is complete surgical excision if symptomatic, but local recurrence rates are as high as 20 % [27].

## Neurogenic Tumors

Neurogenic tumors of the chest wall include neurofibromas and neurilemomas that arise from peripheral nerve sheaths and are usually associated with neurofibromatosis. Presentation is often between the ages of 20 and 30 and are seen as slow growing homogeneous masses on CT and MRI [3]. These lesions may undergo cystic degeneration creating a target appearance on MRI. As one may expect, biopsy is extremely painful. Surgical excision is usually only recommended for cosmetic reasons for cutaneous lesions, as there is a low likelihood of malignancy. However, plexiform lesions that are increasing in size or becoming symptomatic should be completely excised without preoperative biopsy [28].

## Desmoid Tumors

Desmoid tumors arise from musculo-aponeurotic structures and are considered myofibroblastic or fibroblastic in origin. They can develop anywhere in the body, but are most common in the abdomen and extremities, with only 10–28 % arising in the chest wall [1, 10]. The most frequent location in the chest wall being in the shoulder girdle [18]. Their histology is benign, but because of their aggressive growth rates and tendency to grow into nearby structures or cause compressive symptoms, they can be considered malignant. Desmoid tumors are common in females and males, usually younger than 40 years and can be found in patients with familial adenomatous polyposis, where they are related to a mutation in the APC gene. Desmoids can also occur in sites of previous trauma, scar, or radiation. Presentation can consist not only of a palpable chest wall mass/swelling and associated pain, but dyspnea, cough, shortness of breath, and dysphasia have all been reported [18]. The latter symptoms possibly being the result of tumor mass effect. Resection to tumor-free margins is needed for cure, which is difficult to achieve given high incidence of microscopic positive margins [10, 18]. This clearly reinforces the need for wide margins at the time of original resection. Again, appropriate wide excision for a malignant lesion is commonly accepted as full thickness resection with 4-cm margins and en bloc removal of one rib above and below the lesion as well as intercostal muscles, pleura, and wide clear margin of adjacent tissue [17, 18]. When negative margins are not possible, radiation should be considered, though the effectiveness of radiation treatment for nonresectable disease, recurrence, or to treat positive margins, remains with uncertain efficacy [10, 29]. Recurrence rates for desmoid tumor are high. Abbas et al. report 5-year probability of developing a local recurrence as 37 %, with an 89 % rate in patients who had positive margins at the time of resection [17].

### Elastofibromas

Elastofibromas classically occur in the subscapular region, with peak incidence between 40 and 70 years of age. This lesion has a female predominance and a characteristic layered appearance with mild enhancement on CT scan performed with IV contrast [10]. Recommended treatment is complete excision, with intention of cure (Table 8.2).

## Malignant

## Skeletal

Bony malignant chest wall tumors account for 55 % of all chest wall masses and have an average 5-year survival of 60 % [4]. Malignant lesions tend to grow faster, manifest more painfully, and present as larger masses than benign lesions [30]. Primary tumors of the sternum are also usually found to be malignant [3].

### Chondrosarcomas

Chondrosarcomas are most commonly found on the anterior chest wall and account for 30 % of primary malignant bone tumors [31]. They are the most common malignant bony tumor of the chest wall. Chondrosarcomas are rarely found in patients younger than 20 years of age and are found more commonly in a bimodal distribution in the second–third and fourth–fifth decades of life [4, 10, 30]. These tumors represent a malignant degeneration of benign chondromas, with both tumors having similar clinical presentations of painful, hard, slow growing, fixed masses on the anterior chest wall [32]. Additionally, they can be associated with trauma [4]. Radiographic appearance is typically a well-defined mass with soft tissue attenuation associated with cortical destruction, soft tissue attenuation with foci of dense chondroid matrix calcification [2, 6]. Synchronous or metachronous

lung metastases are seen in 10 % of patients at the time of presentation [4]. Pathologic distinction between chondroma and chondrosarocoma is challenging, therefore both tumors are resected with 4-cm margins. Resection is the mainstay of therapy, chemotherapy is largely ineffective, and radiation is reserved for patients who are unresectable or with positive resection margins [10, 32]. Five-year survival is 65–92 %. Tumor-free margin is the largest predictor of local recurrence. Four to ten percent of patients with negative margins will have local recurrence; whereas 73–75 % of those with positive margins will have local recurrence [4, 33].

### Osteosarcomas

Osteosarcomas make up 10–15 % of malignant chest wall tumors, commonly occurring in the rib, scapula, and clavicles [4, 30]. These tumors present as painful masses in young or elderly adults. They often present in the second decade of life [10], specifically cited at puberty in one report [3]. Metastatic disease at the time of presentation is common, with the most common sites being lung, lymph nodes, and liver. The mass appears calcified on imaging with both lytic and calcified or sclerotic osteoid areas [6], and may have hemorrhagic or necrotic components [30]. IV contrast will show areas of different enhancements [6]. Treatment is wide local excision in combination with neoadjuvant chemotherapy. The presence of metastases drastically affects 5-year survival, decreasing it from more than 50 % to between 15 and 20 % [2]. Response to chemotherapy, tumor burden, and presence of metastases are predictive of overall survival [4]. Radiation has been used in cases with an inability to achieve an adequate resection; however, osteosarcomas are not very radiosensitive [10].

### Ewing Sarcoma

The Ewing sarcoma group of tumors is a spectrum of small round-cell tumors that share the chromosomal translocation t(111;22) and include Ewing sarcoma, and primitive neuroectodermal tumor (PNET), which is also known as Askin tumor when located in the chest wall. These tumors are the third most common malignant chest wall tumors overall but are the most common in the pediatric and young adult populations. Males are

**Table 8.2** Benign soft tissue lesions

| Tumor | Origin | Presentation | Imaging characteristics | Treatment |
|---|---|---|---|---|
| Lipomas | Adipose tissue | Well-circumscribed adipose tissue. Found more frequently in older (50–70 yo) and obese patients | Can be difficult to differentiate from low-grade liposarcomas on imaging. Tend to be larger and deeper than at other sites on the body | Excision for symptomatic relief and complete diagnostic analysis |
| Fibromas (desmoid tumors) | Fibrous tissue, myofibroblastic or fibroblastic | Often present <40 yo. Can occur at sites of trauma, scar, radiation, or in pts with familial adenomatous polyposis. Pain, mass, swelling, and sx from mass effect have all been reported | Generally have similar enhancement to muscle. (Variable nondescript appearance depending on collagen content and extent of myxomatous degeneration) | Aggressive growth rates, often resulting in compressive symptoms and tendency to grow into nearby structures. High recurrence rates. Must have resection to tumor-free margin for cure. Radiation tx when negative margins not possible |
| Hemangiomas | Vascular | Painful mass in <30 yo, intramuscular, intercostal, or cavernous | Heterogeneous soft tissue mass with fatty, fibrous, and vascular elements. Ultrasound often used to evaluate flow. MRI can help distinguish between benign and malignant, but surgical biopsy required for definitive diagnosis | Complete surgical excision of symptomatic. High local recurrence rates |
| Neurogenic tumors (neurofibromas, neurilemomas) | Nerve, peripheral nerve sheath tumors | Usually associated with neurofibromatosis. Slow growing. Often occurring between 20 and 30 yo | Homogeneous mass on imaging. May have cystic degeneration creating a target appearance on MRI. Extremely painful if biopsied | Low likelihood of malignancy. Surgical excision of cutaneous lesions for cosmetic reasons. Plexiform lesions that are symptomatic or growing should undergo complete excision |
| Lymphangiomas | Developmental malformation of lymph system | | Cystic or cavernous lesion | Complete surgical excision is standard of care. Treatment with radiation or sclerosing agents=controversial |
| Elastofibroma | | Mass in subscapular region at 40–70 yo, ♀>♂ | CT: characteristic layered appearance with mild enhancement with IV contrast | Local excision is curative |

slightly more affected than females with a 1.6:1 ratio [3]. In addition to the typical chest wall tumor presentation of a painful chest mass, these tumors may also present with systemic symptoms such as fever, malaise, and weight loss, as well as pleural and pericardial effusions [3]. On radiographic imaging, these lesions are often seen as a large noncalcified, soft tissue mass with bone destruction, classically associated with an onion peel or sunburst appearance [3]. They may also have components of hemorrhage or necrosis [6]. The Ewing sarcoma family is an aggressive tumor family with high recurrence rates and high likelihood of metastases [34]. Neoadjuvant chemotherapy is typically given followed by wide local excision with good results. Response to chemotherapy is predictive of local recurrence. Myeloablative therapy and stem cell rescue may improve outcomes in patients with primary metastatic presentation, and bilateral whole-lung radiation has also been used to improve event-free survival with lung, bone, or bone marrow metastasis [3]. While radiation has been shown to provide good local control, it has significant oncogenic potential and cardiopulmonary toxicities in such a young population. Metastases reduce 5-year survival to 30 % from 100 % with local disease at presentation [4].

## Solitary Plasmacytoma

Solitary plasmacytoma is a rare tumor composed of monoclonal plasma cells, as in multiple myeloma; however, this is a discrete mass without diffuse spread. This tumor affects elderly men who present with pain without a mass. Once surgical biopsy has been performed, surgical therapy stops because this tumor is treated primarily with radiation [35]. Five-year survival is 40–60 % and is most dependent on whether or not multiple myeloma develops instead of control of the primary lesion [4]. Two-thirds progress to develop myeloma within 3 years of diagnosis, worsening prognosis, and the rest may achieve permanent cure (Table 8.3).

## Soft Tissue Tumors

Soft tissue tumors commonly present as painless masses, with the anterior chest wall being the most common location for soft tissue malignancies of the thorax [3].

## Soft Tissue Sarcomas

Soft tissue sarcomas are the majority of primary malignant chest wall lesions, but they account for only 6 % of soft tissue sarcomas in the body. They are typically found in middle-aged men who present with a painless mass, except rhabdomyosarcomas, which are more common in children [1]. As with many chest wall tumors, the diagnosis cannot be made radiologically and requires tissue confirmation [15]. The mainstay of treatment is wide local excision. For high-grade sarcomas, 4-cm margins and resection of the rib above and below the lesion is recommended, with reexcision for positive margins [15]. If there is any question about the possibility of full resection, then neoadjuvant therapy should be explored. We will review some of the histologic subtypes later.

## Malignant Fibrous Histiocytomas (MFH)

Malignant fibrous histiocytomas (MFHs) are found in the chest wall but are very common throughout the body, most commonly in the extremities, abdomen, or retroperitoneum. MFH is commonly found in elderly men, and there is usually a history of previous chest wall radiation [36]. Bimodal distribution has also been reported with peaks between 20 and 30 years of age and then again between 50 and 60 years of age [3]. The masses can grow to be a large size but are usually not painful [28]. MFH has a heterogeneous appearance on CT that can be enhancing or calcified, with ill-defined contours [3]. Treatment is wide local excision, and local recurrence rates are higher than 30 % [36]. Pre- and postoperative neoadjuvant chemotherapy are often utilized [37]. Metastatic lesions are diagnosed in 30–50 % of patients, and 5-year survival is only 38 % [28].

## Liposarcomas

Liposarcomas are one of the most common malignant soft tissue tumors in the body, but they are not common in the chest wall [38]. They are rarely found in children and are most common in men ages 40–60 years. It is not unusual for them

**Table 8.3** Malignant bony lesion

| Tumor | Origin | Presentation | Imaging characteristics | Treatment |
|---|---|---|---|---|
| Chondrosarcoma | Cartilage | Anterior chest wall, painful firm mass. Most common malignant bony tumor of chest wall. 30–40 yo. Can be associated with trauma. lung metastasis in 10 % | CT-Well-defined mass with cortical destruction, lobulated soft tissue attenuation with foci of dense chondroid matrix calcification of varied shape and densities | Resection with 4-cm margins. 5-year survival 65–92 % with tumor-free margin. 75 % with + margins → recurrence. Radiation tx for recurrent or unresectable disease |
| Osteosarcoma | Bone | Second most common mal. Chest wall bony tumor. Typically present at puberty, commonly with metastasis | Calcified mass with lytic or sclerotic osteoid bone matrix within the mass. May have hemorrhagic or necrotic components | Wide local excision in combination chemotherapy. Tumor burden, metastasis, and tx response all predict overall survival which ranges from 15 to 50 % |
| Ewing sarcoma family (includes Askin tumor and primitive neuroectodermal tumor) | Bone | Third most common mal. Chest wall tumor overall. Most common in pediatric and young adults, ♂ > ♀ | Large noncalcified, soft tissue mass with bone destruction. May have hemorrhagic or necrotic components. Classically associated with an onion peel or sunburst appearance | Neoadjuvant chemotherapy followed by wide local excision |
| | | | | High recurrence rates and high likelihood of metastasis. Response to chemotherapy predicts recurrence |
| | | | | Myeloablative therapy and stem cell rescue may improve outcomes in patients with metastatic disease |
| Solitary plasmacytoma | Bone marrow/ plasma cells | Rare. Elderly men. Pain without associated mass | Discrete mass without diffuse spread. Needs histologic diagnosis | Radiation. 40–60 % 5 years survival. 2/3 → myeloma. Overall survival is dependent on progression to multiple myeloma |

to be large and frequently associated with trauma. Treatment is wide local excision, and 5-year survival is 60 % [28]. Local recurrence rates are high, and there is little to no role for chemotherapy and radiation.

## Angiosarcoma

Angiosarcoma of the chest wall is a rare vascular tumor that occurs in adults and is associated with chronic lymphedema, irradiation, and chemical exposure [30]. The most common clinical presentation of angiosarcoma of the chest wall is after radiation therapy for breast conservation therapy as part of breast cancer treatment. Patients commonly present 5–10 years after radiation therapy, and 5-year survival after diagnosis is only 16 %

[39]. Wide local excision is the only option for therapy, as most patients cannot have more radiation, and chemotherapy is usually ineffective.

## Rhabdomyosarcoma

Rhabdomyosarcoma is the second most common malignant chest wall tumor in children, following Ewing Sarcoma. It is uncommon to see in adults. Rhabdomyosarcoma is an aggressive tumor with only ~10 % as being fully resectable [3]. Preoperative workup is essential and should include MRI, CT, abdominal US, and bone scan to rule out metastatic disease. Treatment includes pre- and postoperative chemo and radiation therapy in combination with surgical resection (Table 8.4).

**Table 8.4** Malignant soft tissue lesions

| Tumor | Origin | Presentation | Imaging characteristics | Treatment/prognosis |
|---|---|---|---|---|
| Soft tissue sarcomas (liposarcomas, synovial sarcomas, rhabdomyosarcomas, fibrosarcoma, neurofibrosarcoma) | Any soft tissue (adipose, synovium, muscle, fibrous tissue, nerve) | Majority of primary malignant chest wall lesions. Middle-aged men with painless mass (exception: Rhabdomyosarcoma = most common in children) | Heterogeneous appearance with varying levels of enhancement and calcification depending on the histology | Wide local excision with 4-cm margins and rib above and below for high-grade lesions. Reexcision for + margins or recurrent disease. Most = poor prognosis with survival influenced by histology, tumor grade, tumor burden, and location |
| Malignant Fibrous Histiocytomas (MFH) | Fibrous tissue | Elderly men, usually with history of prior chest radiation, usually not painful, but may become large | CT: heterogeneous appearance enhancing or calcified with ill-defined contours | Neoadjuvant chemotherapy followed by wide local excision and further chemotherapy. Local recurrence >30%. 5 years survival 38% |
| Liposarcoma | Adipose tissue | Men ages 40–60 yo, may be associated with trauma | | Wide local excision. 5 years survival 60% High local recurrence rates |
| Neurofibrosarcomas (malignant schwannomas or malignant peripheral nerve sheath tumors) | Nerve | Associated with radiation, neurofibromitosis (29% will develop this tumor) [3]. Men 40–50 yo, painful mass | | Wide local excision and postoperative radiation. 5-years survival=55% [28] |
| Rhabdomyosarcoma | Muscle | Second most common malignant chest wall tumor in children. Uncommon in adults | | Pre- and postoperative neoadjuvant chemo and radiotherapy combined with surgical resection. Aggressive tumors with only 10% fully resectable |
| Fibrosarcoma | Fibrous tissue | | Heterogeneous masses on CT and MRI may have areas of necrosis and hemorrhage | Neoadjuvant chemotherapy followed by resection. Postoperative radiation used if margins +. Likely to have local recurrence and/or metastasize |
| Angiosarcoma | Vascular | Associated with chronic lymphedema, irradiation, and chemical exposure. Most commonly 5–10 years after radiation tx for breast cancer | | Wide local excision. 5-years survival 16%. Not candidates for further radiation. Chemotherapy is ineffective |

## Radiation-Associated Malignant Tumors and Metastatic Disease

Radiation-associated malignant tumors of the chest wall are uncommon but not rare [1]. Cancers of the breast and lung or lymphomas are common indications for radiation to the chest. In a large series from Memorial Sloan-Kettering Cancer Center, in 361 patients, 21 (6 %) chest wall tumors arose in patients with a history of radiation to the chest. These patients were all treated with resection and had similar survival as that of patients with tumors arising de novo [40].

Not all chest wall tumors are primary lesions. Metastatic lesions from breast, lung, or unknown primary tumors can be found in the chest wall, and the role for surgical resection is gaining clarity. In the case of unknown primaries, chest wall lesions are treated like a primary tumor with resection for tissue diagnosis and therapy [41]. For breast cancers, formal studies are still lacking, but one large series from Chicago found an increase in survival with control of a chest wall lesion with either surgery or radiation [37]. Chest wall and sternal resection for metastatic cancers is associated with relief of pain from ulceration and bleeding caused by disease recurrence (Fig. 8.5).

## Pediatric Tumors

Like tumors in their adult counterparts, pediatric chest wall tumors are varied in their histology, presentation, and age of onset; however, they have their own diagnostic and therapeutic challenges [42]. Approximately 20 % of chest tumors in childhood are located in the chest wall, and histologic diagnoses can range from benign to malignant and infectious to noninfectious [43]. There is also wide variability in incidence of disease by country. In underdeveloped countries, tuberculosis of the chest wall is more prevalent than the common North American malignancies to which we are more accustomed. Ewing sarcoma is the most common malignant diagnosis in children vs. chondrosarcomas in adults [44].

Because of the young age of pediatric patients, both survival data and long-term effects of treatment have to be considered in multidisciplinary treatment planning. Chemotherapy and aggres-sive surgical resection are the mainstays of therapy with a goal to avoid radiation therapy where possible. Preoperative chemotherapy is given to most chemosensitive tumors to allow for improved local control, less extensive surgery, and to treat micrometastatic disease. Scoliosis, restrictive pulmonary function, hypoplasia of soft tissues, and secondary tumors are some of the long-term sequelae that can be seen in children after treatment of a chest wall tumor [44].

## Surgical Management

Chest wall resection is the primary treatment modality for chest wall tumors and can be performed with low morbidity and mortality. If tumors are chemosensitive, preoperative chemotherapy should be administered to reduce the tumor burden. Osteosarcoma, rhabdomyosarcoma, Ewing sarcoma, and other small-cell sarcomas should be treated with chemotherapy in a neoadjuvant setting, and then continued postoperatively depending on tumor response. Chondrosarcomas and other adult soft tissue sarcomas are typically excised surgically and irradiated if negative margins cannot be achieved. Resection can prolong survival and provide palliation for symptomatic lesions [45].

Extent of tumor location and invasion may influence preoperative planning and intraoperative approach. Depending on the extent of pulmonary involvement, a double lumen endotracheal tube may be required to allow for concurrent pulmonary resection. In one review of 25 years of data, 34 % of chest wall tumors infiltrated into the lung, requiring associated lung resection [12]. Placing a thoracoscope in the chest, away from the lesion, may be useful to determine extent of pulmonary involvement and exact location when the lesion is not palpable. When necessary, a needle can be inserted into the chest under thoracoscopic guidance to aid in operative planning. Appropriate margins are dependent on the histology of the tumor and are a key predictor of recurrence-free survival [46]. For aggressive malignancies that can spread along the periosteum, the entire rib should be resected with costal articulations either posteriorly or anteriorly depending on tumor location. Sections of ribs above and below the tumor

**Fig. 8.5** Resected metastatic colon cancer to rib

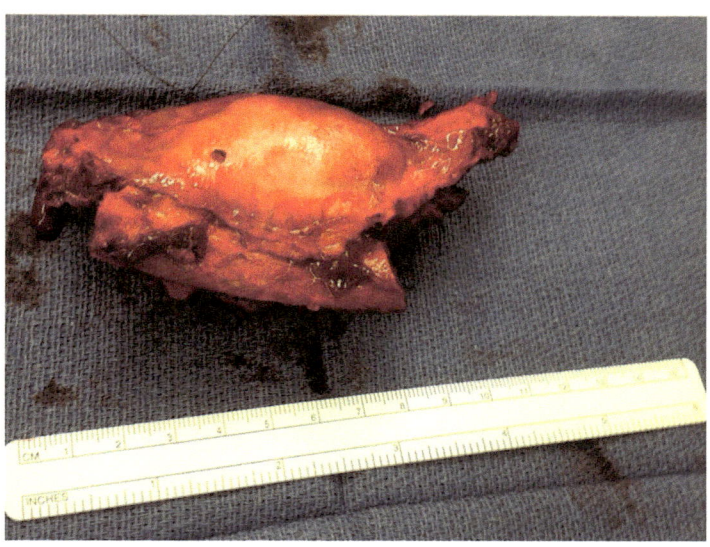

should be resected as well. For high-grade malignancies, 4-cm margins are adequate, and low-grade malignancies can be treated with 1–2 cm margins. Desmoid tumors are not technically malignant, but their behavior is so aggressive that one should use 4-cm margins for these lesions when possible. Any involved soft tissue, skin, underlying pleura, or lung tissue should be resected with the tumor, provided pulmonary function permits resection.

Adequate oncologic resection should not be compromised for concern over chest wall defect; however, the integrity of the chest wall should be maintained to avoid pulmonary compromise.

## Reconstruction

Chest wall reconstruction after large en bloc resection is often accomplished as part of a multidisciplinary team in conjunction with plastic surgery. The choice of material and method of reconstruction largely depends on anatomic location and surgeon preference. Goals of reconstructive therapy include preserving respiratory and body mechanics, visceral protection, and cosmetic outcome.

*The main tenants of chest wall reconstruction are as follows* [2]:

1. Defects less than 4–5 cm typically do not require reconstruction.
2. Posterior defects covered by the scapula do not require reconstruction.
3. Defects located at the scapular tip must be reconstructed to prevent the scapula from becoming trapped within the defect.
4. Skeletal stabilization is achieved with autologous tissue, mesh, Gore-Tex (W.L. gore and Associates, Inc. Flagstaff, AZ) or methyl methacrylate "sandwich" reconstruction.
5. Soft tissue reconstruction can be performed using myocutaneous or omental flaps.

Autologous tissue flaps can be constructed from a variety of soft tissue donor sites, including: the Latissimus dorsi, Pectoralis Major, Rectus Abdominal muscle flap (VRAM or TRAM), External obliques, Trapezius, or Omentum flap. The specifics and details of these reconstructions are beyond the scope of this chapter. As mentioned previously, it is important to keep in mind location of the defect, locations, and types of prior

**Fig. 8.6** Chest wall reconstruction of the fifth rib space using a gortex patch in a patient with prior chest wall resection and gortex patch reconstruction for desmoid tumor of the chest wall

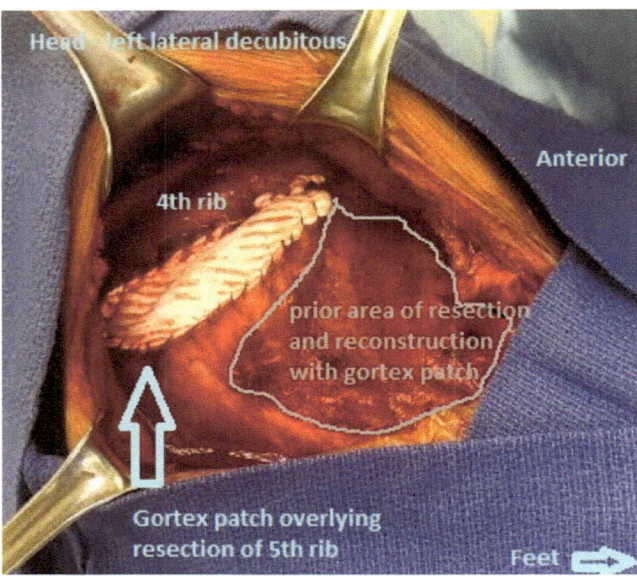

surgical procedures, prior oncologic history and treatment, or any prior areas of radiation when choosing a suitable donor site for soft tissue reconstruction (Fig. 8.6).

Reconstruction in pediatric patients can be challenging given ongoing growth of the chest wall and intrathoracic components. Large resections and reconstructions often leave chest wall asymmetry despite reconstructive efforts. This asymmetry can become more pronounced as the child grows and may lead to the development of skeletal deformities such as scoliosis [15]. Children should continue to undergo long-term follow-up while growing, with specific attention to chest wall development and associated bony abnormalities including scoliosis screening.

## Postoperative Management

In the immediate postoperative period, use of epidural catheters or localized infusion catheters for pain control can minimize postoperative morbidity and mortality. Largely because of increased ability to engage in and adequately perform appropriate pulmonary hygiene. Postoperative pulmonary hygiene is vitally important because large anterior

defects can result in weak cough and inability to clear secretions, leading to debilitating pneumonia. Bronchoscopy may be necessary to facilitate adequate pulmonary hygiene in these patients.

## Surveillance

Duration and frequency of postoperative surveillance will vary depending on age of the patient, tumor type, presentation, stage, response to treatment, and ability to obtain clean margins at the time of surgical resection.

## Summary

Chest wall tumors are a heterogeneous group of lesions that provide an interesting diagnostic and therapeutic challenge for surgeons. Careful preoperative evaluation of the patient, radiographic imaging, and histopathology are required. In general, treatment is wide local excision, with margins for malignant disease being wider (4-cm margins when possible), and adjuvant radiation is typically given in the event of positive margins. Local control is the most important prognostic factor, with disease-free survival for malignant disease being limited by positive margins. Chemotherapy is rarely effective, but may be helpful as neoadjuvant therapy prior to resection in the event of large tumor burden. For advanced disease or lesions that may result in significant functional loss, multidisciplinary preoperative planning is indicated, involving thoracic surgery, plastic surgery, neurosurgery, radiation medicine, oncology, and physical medicine and rehabilitation. Excellent outcomes for patients with benign, primary malignant, and metastatic lesions of the chest wall can be obtained with complete surgical resection and appropriate reconstruction.

# References

1. Park BJ, Flores RM. Chest wall tumors. In: Shields TW, Locicero J, Reed CE, Feins RH, editors. General thoracic surgery. Philadelphia: Lippincott; 2009. p. 669–78.
2. David E, Marshall M. Review of chest wall tumors: a diagnostic, therapeutic, and reconstructive challenge. Semin Plast Surg. 2011;25:16–24.
3. Smith SE, Keshavjee S. Primary chest wall tumors. Thorac Surg Clin. 2010;20:495–507.
4. Shah AA, D'Amico TA. Primary chest wall tumors. J Am Coll Surg. 2010;210:360–6.
5. Tateishi U, Gladish GW, Kusumoto M, et al. Chest wall tumors: radiologic findings and pathologic correlation: part1. Benign tumors. Radiographics. 2003;23:1477–90.
6. Rocca M, et al. The role of imaging for the surgeon in primary malignant bone tumors of the chest wall. Eur J Radiol. 2013;82:2070–5.
7. Lee TJ, Collins J. MR imaging evaluation of disorders of the chest wall. Magn Reson Imaging Clin N Am. 2008;16:355–79. x.
8. Carter BW, Gladish GW. MR imaging of chest wall tumors. Magn Reson Imaging Clin N Am. 2015;23:197–215.
9. Incarbone M, Pastorino U. Surgical treatment of chest wall tumors. World J Surg. 2001;25:218–30.
10. Kim JY, Hofstetter WL. Tumors of the mediastinum and chest wall. Surg Clin North Am. 2010;90:1019–40.
11. Petermann D, Allenbach G, Schmidt S, et al. Value of positron emission tomography in full-thickness chest wall resections for malignancies. Interact Cardiovasc Thorac Surg. 2009;9:406.
12. Caroli G, et al. Accuracy of transthoracic ultrasound for the prediction of chest wall infiltration by lung cancer and of lung infiltration by chest wall tumors. Heart Lung Circ. 2015;24:1–7. http://dx.doi.org/10.1016/j.hlc.2015.03.018

13. Kucharczuk JC, Kaiser LR. Chest wall resections. In: Kaiser LR, Kron IL, Spray TL, editors. Mastery of cardiothoracic surgery. Philadelphia: Lippincott; 2007. p. 222–7.
14. Tomo H, Ito Y, Aono M, Takaoka K. Chest wall deformity associated with osteochondroma of the scapula: a case report and review of the literature. J Shoulder Elbow Surg. 2005;14:103–6.
15. Dingemann C, et al. Thoracic wall reconstruction for primary malignancies in children: short- and long-term results. Eur J Pediatr Surg. 2012;22:34–9.
16. Shackcloth MJ, Page RD. Scapular osteochondroma with reactive bursitis presenting as a chest wall tumour. Eur J Cardiothorac Surg. 2000;18:495–6.
17. Abbas AE, Deschamps C, Cassivi SD, et al. Chest-wall desmoid tumors: results of surgical intervention. Ann Thorac Surg. 2004;78:1219–23. discussion 1219-1223.
18. Matrai Z, et al. Sporadic desmoid tumors of the chest: long-term follow-up of 28 multimodally treated patients. Eur J Cardiothorac Surg. 2011;40:1170–6.
19. Eroglu A, Kurkcuoglu IC, Karaoglanoglu N. Solitary eosinophilic granuloma of sternum. Ann Thorac Surg. 2004;77:329–31.
20. Bayram AS, Koprucuoglu M, Filiz G, Gebitekin C. Case of solitary eosinophilic granuloma of the sternum. Thorac Cardiovasc Surg. 2008;56:117–8.
21. Biswas S, Keddington J. Soft right chest wall swelling simulating lipoma following motor vehicle accident: transdiaphragmatic intercostal hernia. A case report and review of literature. Hernia. 2008;12:539–43.
22. Takamori S, Miwa K, Hayashi A, Shirouzu K. Intramuscular lipoma in the chest wall. Eur J Cardiothorac Surg. 2004;26:1038.
23. Ozpolat B, Ozeren M, Akkaya T, Yucel E. Giant lipoma of chest wall. Eur J Cardiothorac Surg. 2004;26:437.
24. Eren S, Avci A. Giant cystic lymphangioma in the thoracic wall in a newborn. Asian Cardiovasc Thorac Ann. 2009;17:659.
25. Yildirim E, Dural K, Kaplan T, Sakinci U. Cystic lymphangioma: report of two atypical cases. Interact Cardiovasc Thorac Surg. 2004;3:63–5.
26. Sakurai K, Hara M, Ozawa Y, Nakagawa M, Shibamoto Y. Thoracic hemangioma: imagining via CT, MR and PET along with pathologic correlation. J Thorac Imaging. 2008;23:114–20.
27. Griffo S, Stassano P, De Luca G, Di Tommaso L, Monaco M, Spiezia S. Intramuscular hemangioma of the chest wall: an unusual tumor. J Thorac Cardiovasc Surg. 2007;134:1368–9.
28. Gallo AE, Coady MA. Chest wall tumors. In: Yuh DD, Vricella LA, Baumgartner WA, editors. The Johns Hopkins manual of cardiothoracic surgery. New York: McGraw Hill; 2007. p. 75–90.
29. Bolke E, Krasniqi H, Lammering G, et al. Chest wall and intrathoracic desmoid tumors: surgical experience and review of the literature. Eur J Med Res. 2009;14:240–3.
30. Tateishi U, Gladish GW, Kusumoto M, et al. Chest wall tumors: radiologic findings and pathologic cor-

relation: part 2. Malignant tumors. Radiographics. 2003;23:1491–508. Review.

31. Stanic V, Vulovic T, Novakovic M, et al. Radical resection of giant chondrosarcoma of the anterior chest wall. Vojnosanit Pregl. 2008;65:64–8.

32. Somers J, Faber LP. Chondroma and chondrosarcoma. Semin Thorac Cardiovasc Surg. 1999;11:270–7.

33. Widhe B, Bauer HCF, Scandinavian Sarcoma Group. Surgical treatment is decisive for outcome in chondrosarcoma of the chest wall: a population-based Scandinavian Sarcoma Group study of 106 patients. J Thorac Cardiovasc Surg. 2009;137:610–4.

34. Lee WS, Kim YH, Chee HK, et al. Multimodal treatment of primary extra skeletal Ewing's sarcoma of the chest wall: report of 2 cases. Cancer Res Treat. 2009;41:108–12.

35. Bousnina S, Zendah I, Marniche K, et al. Solitary plasmocytoma of the rib: a rare tumor not to miss. Rev Pneumol Clin. 2006;62:243–6.

36. Yoshida N, Miyanari N, Yamamoto Y, Egami H. Successful treatment of malignant fibrous histiocytoma originating in the chest wall: report of a case. Surg Today. 2006;36:714–21.

37. Hazard HW, Gorla SR, Scholtens D, Kiel K, Gradishar WJ, Khan SA. Surgical resection of the primary tumor, chest wall control, and survival in women with metastatic breast cancer. Cancer. 2008;113:2011–9.

38. Shoji T, Sonobe M, Okubo K, Wada H, Bando T, Date H. Giant primary liposarcoma of the chest. Gen Thorac Cardiovasc Surg. 2009;57:159–61.

39. Styring E, Fernebro J, Jonsson PE, et al. Changing clinical presentation of angiosarcomas after breast cancer: from late tumors in edematous arms to earlier tumors on the thoracic wall. Breast Cancer Res Treat. 2010;122:883–7.

40. Schwarz RE, Burt M. Radiation-associated malignant tumors of the chest wall. Ann Surg Oncol. 1996;3:387–92.

41. Haraguchi S, Hioki M, Takushima M, Yanagimoto K, Koizumi K, Shimizu K. Metastatic chest wall tumor suspected to be of lung origin by immunoreactivity for cytokeratin 7 and 20. Jpn J Thorac Cardiovasc Surg. 2006;54:132–6.

42. La Quaglia MP. Chest wall tumors in child hood and adolescence. Semin Pediatr Surg. 2008;17:173–80.

43. Wyttenbach R, Vock P, Tschappeler H. Cross-sectional imaging with CT and/or MRI of pediatric chest tumors. Eur Radiol. 1998;8:1040–6.

44. van den Berg H, van Rijn RR, Merks JHM. Management of tumors of the chest wall in childhood: a review. J Pediatr Hematol Oncol. 2008;30:214–21.

45. Ryan MB, McMurtrey MJ, Roth JA. Current management of chest-wall tumors. Surg Clin North Am. 1989;69:1061–80.

46. King RM, Pairolero PC, Trastek VF, Piehler JM, Payne WS, Bernatz PE. Primary chest wall tumors: factors affecting survival. Ann Thorac Surg. 1986;41:597–601.

# Role of Nurse Practitioners in Chest Wall Clinics as a Model for Care

Mary Zanobini, Barbara Goebel, Amy B. Powne, Robyn H. Lao, and Karen S. Brand

Pectus excavatum, pectus carinatum, and rib resections are common chest wall deformities requiring surgical correction during the pediatric and adolescent period. The Ravitch and Nuss procedures are common surgical operations to treat these anterior chest wall deformities. Rib resections can be performed for oncological diagnostic purposes or to treat high-risk rib fractures. Nursing care focused on preoperative teaching as well as postoperative pain management is integral to successful outcomes for patients undergoing these procedures [1]. In addition, nursing interventions should address the patients' emotional and psychological well-being regarding their chest wall deformity.

M. Zanobini, N.P., R.N.F.A. (✉)
B. Goebels, N.P., R.N.F.A.
Pediatric Heart Center, University of California, Davis Children's Hospital, 2315 Stockton Blvd., Suite 7133, Sacramento, CA, USA
e-mail: mfzanobini@ucdavis.edu

A. Powne, R.N., C.N.S. • R.H. Lao, R.N., M.S.N., D.N.P., C.P.N.P.-AC.
University of California, Davis Children's Hospital, Sacramento, CA, USA

K.S. Brand, R.N., M.S.N., C.P.N.P.-AC.
Shriners Hospital of Northern California, Sacramento, CA, USA

## Nursing Care

### Pectus Excavatum

Pectus excavatum is the most common congenital chest wall deformity and is characterized by posterior depression of the sternum and adjacent costal cartilages. The cause of pectus excavatum is unclear [2, 3]. Initially, a parent will notice a chest wall defect immediately after birth and this may cause some concern. Parents should be reassured that chest wall defects do not cause young children any harm and can be monitored throughout the child's growth spurts until the early teenage years. Pectus excavatum may increase during periods of rapid growth. As the child matures, the appearance of their chest often causes stress related to altered body image [4]. Parents and children should be reassured that pectus excavatum does not cause any damage to the underlying lungs or heart. Affected children may experience chest pain or shortness of breath with exercise [5]. They may have trouble competing with their peers during a sport involving physical exertion [6]. An echocardiogram may show mitral valve or tricuspid regurgitation or mitral valve prolapse. These are often reasons why a family will seek help from a health care provider. Many times correction of pectus excavatum is not covered by health insurance providing added stress to the family.

© Springer International Publishing Switzerland 2017
G.W. Raff, S. Hirose (eds.), *Surgery for Chest Wall Deformities*,
DOI 10.1007/978-3-319-43926-6_9

Psychosocial concerns: Concern about the appearance of the chest prompts many, if not most, patients to have the chest wall deformity corrected. A large percentage of pectus excavatum patients are self-conscious about their chests. Children and adolescents with potentially visible physical differences may be at risk for body image and interpersonal difficulties [4].

The most common corrective surgery for pectus excavatum is a Nuss procedure where a metal (nickel or titanium) bar is inserted behind the sternum [2]. If a nickel allergy is suspected, a titanium bar will be used. The Nuss procedure can be quite painful. More recently, the use of cryoablation has significantly decreased pain associated with the Nuss Bar procedure. Historically, hospital stay for a patient receiving a Nuss Bar has been 7–10 days, mainly for pain control. With effective cryoablation, patients are being discharged in 2–3 days postoperatively and requiring considerably less opioid narcotics.

Cryoablation of the pectoral nerves is very effective for pain control and may last up to 12 weeks postoperatively. Cryoablation is a mechanism in which Nitrous Oxide (N2O) is used to cool a probe that will rapidly extract heat from the intercostal nerve bundle causing the nerve to freeze. Within 24–48 h, the stunned nerve bundle will temporarily cease to transmit pain for up to 12 weeks. The affected nerves axons will regenerate and nerve function will resume over several weeks.

A patient may have a mixed chest wall deformity consisting of pectus excavatum and pectus carinatum (protrusion of the sternum and ribs) and the surgeon may recommend the Ravitch procedure.

The goal of the Ravitch procedure is to remove abnormal rib cartilage while preserving the perichondrium, allowing regrowth of rib cartilage to the sternum in a more anatomic fashion [7]. Other key elements in the operation include performing a sternal osteotomy to allow redirection of the sternum and stabilization of the sternum with a metal bar, when necessary [7].

## Preoperative Preparation for the Nuss Procedure or the Ravitch Procedure

Chest CT will be used to measure a Haller index. A Haller index over 3.2 is an indication for corrective surgery [8].

Pulmonary function tests are helpful to anesthesiologists for lung capacity and also for comparison pre- and postoperatively of lung function.

Echocardiogram should be carried out to identify any heart defects such as mitral valve regurgitation or prolapse and tricuspid regurgitation associated with pectus excavatum.

AP and lateral chest X-rays are ordered for pre- and postoperative comparison. Photographs may be taken for the same reason.

Timing of surgery: Ideally, the pectus repair will be performed before the end of adolescence. Logistically, planning surgery in the summer months can be less disruptive to the patients sporting and educational activities.

Patient and family should be prepared for a hospital length of stay anywhere between 2 and 10 days depending on modalities used for pain control.

Timing of surgery: Ideally, the pectus repair will be performed before the end of adolescence. Logistically, planning surgery in the summer months can be less disruptive to the patients sporting and educational activities.

## Postoperative Care Following the Nuss or the Ravitch Procedure

### Immediate Postoperative Period

Often patients are admitted to the intensive care unit over 24–48 h for close observation of respiratory status and pain control.

### Pulmonary

Chest tube to suction pressure of 20 cm water is commonly used to assist with drainage of effusions or air caused by surgery to the chest cavity.

Initially, aggressive pulmonary toilet is required to prevent postoperative atelectasis often intermittent positive pressure breathing every 4 h by a respiratory therapist and incentive spirometry every hour is encouraged by nursing.

Monitoring of oxygen saturations is important during the immediate postoperative period and oxygen via nasal cannula may be necessary for shallow breathing associated with chest discomfort.

Chest X-rays are taken immediately postoperatively before discharge for comparison and to identify pleural effusions or a pneumothorax which may occur as a consequence of the Nuss procedure.

## Cardiac and Hemodynamics

An arterial line may be placed for the first 24 h to monitor blood pressure and heart rate; this may be removed in 24 h if the patient is hemodynamically stable.

Maintenance intravenous fluids will be necessary until the patient can tolerate oral fluids.

Foley catheter to monitor urine output may be recommended for 24 h postoperatively.

## Pain Control

This procedure can be very painful and monitoring of pain levels with adequate pain medication is paramount for patient mobility and recovery.

Many surgeons will use cryoablation as a pectoral nerves block which will take effect in 24–48 h and last up to 12 weeks for thoracic pain management.

Dilaudid or Morphine PCA is often used dimmediately postoperatively. In addition, a local anesthetic with an On Q pump containing Ropivacaine for continuous local infusion may be necessary until the cyroablation of the pectoral nerves becomes effective in 12–24 hours.

Muscle spasm can be controlled with diazepam. Ketorolac, an intravenous nonsteroidal anti-inflammatory, may also augment pain control.

Neurontin at bedtime for 3–6 months postoperatively is helpful for neuropathic pain or paresthesia related to cryoablation.

Oral pain medication may be started and intravenous medications weaned when the patient can tolerate a regular diet. Percocet or Norco with scheduled Naproxen or ibuprofen is often effective.

## Gastrointestinal

Oral fluids and a regular diet can be initiated as soon as the patient can tolerate them on the evening of surgery or the next morning. A histamine H2-receptor antagonist such as Zantac may be useful until a regular diet is established.

A bowel regime using Miralax, Colace, Senna orally and Bisocodyl suppository is recommended while the patient needs narcotic medication.

## Activity

The patient should get out of bed to a chair the evening of surgery or the next morning. Strict log rolling is advised to avoid bar displacement and the patient should not push down through their arms or twist their upper body while getting up for the same reason. The patient is encouraged not to slouch which is intuitive for patients with pectus excavatum and the patient should not raise their arms above their head. Ambulation is encouraged on postoperative day 1, gradually increasing time out of bed.

## Discharge and Follow-Up

Patients are discharged home when pain is controlled by oral medication and a regular diet and fluids are tolerated. Prescriptions for pain control and prevention of constipation are recommended as well as Diazepam and Neurontin for muscle spasm and nerve pain/paresthesia.

Surgical wounds are closed with dissolvable sutures and either Dermabond or Steri-strips. It is okay to shower once the patient has been discharged home and gently clean the incision sites with soap and water, then pat dry with a towel. No swimming, wading, or soaking in a bathtub for the first month. No lotions, salves, powders, ointments, or cream/paste on the wounds. For the first month after surgery it is recommended that the patient not to do any strenuous activities. No slouching or slumping while sitting up and when bending over it is important to bend at the hip. Good posture helps keep the Nuss bar in place.

Activity restrictions for 3 months postoperatively include: no twisting, no weight bearing on arms to change position, no lifting arms above head, no running, no jumping, no pivoting, no sit-ups, no swimming, no heavy lifting, and no contact sports. Specifically, no karate, judo, gymnastics, golf, or contact sports for the first 3 months. It is important to remind the patient that no heavy lifting for the first 3 months includes no backpacks full of schoolbooks. As a general rule, if it weighs more than a gallon of milk it is too heavy. Frequent walking is encouraged. Letters for accommodations for school should be provided for two sets of books and extra time to travel between classes. No Physical Education class for 3 months. With effective cryoablation, patients frequently forget they have had a bar placed in their chest and need to be reminded of the physical restrictions..

Follow-up in clinic should be scheduled for 2–4 weeks for wound check and then in 3 months, 6 months, 1 year, and 2 years, postoperatively. CXR may be taken as needed for postoperative monitoring. Photographs of the chest may be taken once postoperatively to record positive effects of surgery.

The most common early complications are wound problems and bar displacement.

A letter may be provided for air travel and future need for MRI related to a metal bar inserted into the chest. MRI examinations can be performed, however, the bar may cause artifact if the MRI is of the chest or upper abdomen.

After 2–3 years the surgeon will remove the Nuss bar which is a same day surgery procedure. Research shows that surgical repair of pectus excavatum has a positive impact on both the physical and psychosocial well-being of the child [9].

## Pectus Carinatum

Pectus Carinatum is a spectrum of protrusion abnormalities of the anterior chest wall [10].

## Management

Patients with pectus carinatum can be managed with bracing as young as 8–10 years old. Thoracic bracing will help to mold the shape of the chest as the child grows and while the chest wall is compliant.

The patient is initially examined in the chest wall clinic and deemed a good candidate for bracing. This form of treatment must be agreed upon by the patient, parents, and physician because the child will have to wear the brace up to 20–22 h a day for a positive change in the shape to the chest.

A chest brace is made for each individual patient according to the need for chest molding using 3D imaging.

The child is monitored closely when the brace is new. Initial clinic visits involve checking the skin under the brace for breakdown. The family may be encouraged to apply rubbing alcohol to the skin of the chest to prevent skin breakdown and improve patients comfort level. A thin t-shirt should be worn under the brace. When the brace is picked up initially the skin is carefully checked for erythema. There should be some areas of mild erythema over the chest protrusions; this indicates the mold has been made appropriately. The child should be encouraged to wear the brace initially for 20 min at a time and removing the brace to allow erythema to subside and prevent skin breakdown. Time in the brace can be increased to 1 h then 2 h and gradually to 6 h at a time. Once the brace has been worn effectively for 6 h, the child may start to sleep in the brace. The objective is to have the child wear the brace for 20 h a day. Initially, sleeping in the brace is difficult but the child quickly gets used to being able to sleep in the brace. The brace is removed for sports and showering.

Patients are monitored in the clinic every 3–6 months while in the bracing program. Effective bracing for pectus carinatum is dependent on the child wearing the brace. Serial photographs are useful for monitoring changes in the shape of the chest wall.

## Rib Resection

A rib resection is the surgical removal of a segment of a rib or ribs. Rib resections are performed to treat fractures that are at risk for damaging lung tissue, to remove sections of rib damaged by diseases such as cancer, or to obtain bone for a bone graft.

Thoracic outlet syndrome results from the compression of blood vessels or nerve fibers between the neck and the axilla. A rib resection can be part of the treatment plan for thoracic outlet syndrome [11].

The site of the surgical incision will depend not only on the location of the rib to be removed, but also on the nature of any additional surgical procedures.

Ribs are attached to the spine, and the upper ribs also attach to the sternum. For this reason, rib sections used for bone grafting are most easily obtained from the lowest rib, which remains free floating in the front of the rib cage.

## Preoperative Preparation

Pre-op appointment will include a complete history and physical, an AP and lateral chest X-ray, and basic lab work. These are the minimal tests required for a thoracic surgery.

## Intraoperative

Surgical approach will be determined by the location of the affected rib. Typically, the rib resection will be done via a right or left thoracotomy which allows access into the thoracic cavity. General anesthesia with intubation is required. Often, intercostal nerve blocks are performed before closing the thoracotomy incision for optimal pain control.

## Postoperative Care Following a Rib Resection

### Immediate Postoperative Period

Often patients are admitted to the intensive care unit for 24–48 h for close observation of respiratory status and pain control.

Chest tube to suction pressure of 20 cm water is commonly used to assist with drainage of effusions or air caused by surgery to the chest cavity.

Aggressive pulmonary toilet is required to prevent postoperative atelectasis often intermittent positive pressure breathing q 4 hourly by respiratory therapist and incentive spirometry every hour is encouraged by nursing.

Monitoring of oxygen saturations is important during the immediate postoperative period and oxygen via nasal cannula may be necessary for shallow breathing associated with chest discomfort.

Chest X-rays are taken postoperatively to identify pleural effusions or a pneumothorax which may occur as a consequence of the thoracotomy and rib resection procedure.

### Cardiac and Hemodynamics

An arterial line may be placed for the first 24 h to monitor blood pressure and heart rate; this may be removed in 24 h if the patient is hemodynamically stable.

Maintenance intravenous fluids will be necessary until the patient can tolerate oral fluids.

Foley catheter to monitor urine output may be recommended for 24 h postoperatively.

### Pain Control

This procedure can be very painful and monitoring of pain levels with adequate pain medication is paramount for patient mobility and recovery.

Many surgeons will use intercostal nerves blocks and cryoablation to optimize pain control. In addition, intravenous narcotics may be used to help with initial pain control.

## Gastrointestinal

Oral fluids and a regular diet can be initiated as soon as the patient can tolerate them on the evening of surgery or the next morning. A histamine H2-receptor antagonist such as Zantac IV/po may be useful until a regular diet is established.

A bowel regime using Miralax, Colace, Senna orally and Bisocodyl suppository is recommended while the patient needs narcotic medication.

## Activity

The patient should get out of bed to a chair the evening of surgery or the next morning. Ambulation is encouraged on postoperative day 1 gradually increasing time out of bed.

## Discharge and Follow-Up

Patients are discharged home when pain is controlled by oral medication and regular diet and fluids are tolerated. Prescriptions for pain control and prevention of constipation are recommended.

Surgical wounds are closed with dissolvable sutures and possibly Dermabond. A shower is okay but no bathing or swimming or hot tub for 2 weeks until the incision is well healed.

Activity restrictions: for the first 2 weeks, no strenuous or vigorous activities and the incision heels.

Follow-up in clinic should be scheduled for 1–2 weeks for wound check. Additional follow-up will be determined based on indication for the rib resection.

## References

1. Roskos PL, Conlon PM, Blazejak DL, Siebrecht AL. Improving care of patients following minimally invasive pectus excavatum repair with standardization and collaboration. J Pediatr Surg Nurs. 2016;5(1):22–7.
2. Frantz F. Indications and guidelines for pectus excavatum repair. Curr Opin Pediatr. 2011;23:486–91.
3. Goretxky MJ, Kelly Jr RE, Croitoru D, Nuss D. Chest wall anomalies: pectus excavatum and pectus carinatum. Adolesc Med Clin. 2004;15(3):455–7.
4. Einsidel R, Clausner A. Funnel chest, psycological and psychomatic aspects in children, youngsters and young adults. J Cardiovasc Surg. 1999;40(5):733–6.
5. Koumbourlis AC. Pectus excavatum: pathophysiology and clinical characteristics. Paediatr Respir Rev. 2009;10(1):3–6.
6. Jaroszewski D, Ntorica D, McMahon L, Steidley E, Deschamps C. Current management of pectus excavatum: a review and update of therapy and treatment recommendations. J Am Board Fam Med. 2010;23(2):230–9.
7. Ravitch MM. The operative treatment of pectus excavatum. Ann Surg. 1948;4(129):429–44.
8. Kelly RE, Goretsky MJ, Obermeyer R, Kuhn MA, Redlinger R, Janey TS, Moskowitz A, Nuss D. Twenty-one years of experience with minimally invasive repair of pectus excavatum by the Nuss procedure in 1215 patients. Ann Surg. 2010;252(6):1072–81.
9. Lawson ML, Cash TF, Akers RA, Vasser E, Burke B, Tabangin M, et al. A pilot study of the impact of surgical repair on disease-specific quality of life among patients with pectus excavatum. J Pediatr Surg. 2003;38:916–8.
10. Fonkalsrud EW, Anselmo DM. Less extensive techniques for repair of pectus carinatum: the undertreated chest deformity. J Am Coll Surg. 2004;198(6):898–905.
11. Orlando MS, Likes KC, Mirza S, Cao Y, Cohen A, Lum YW, et al. A decade of excellent outcomes after surgical intervention in 538 patients with thoracic outlet syndrome. J Am Coll Surg. 2014;5(220):934–9.

# Index

**A**

Accessory muscles, 5
Acellular dermal matrices (ADM), 63
ADM. *See* Acellular dermal matrices (ADM)
Analgesic adjuncts
α2-adrenoceptor agonists, 38
gabapentinoids, 38–39
ketamine, 38
magnesium, 39
Anesthesia, 39–41
α2-adrenoceptor, 34
airway management, 36
anxiety, 34
benzodiazepines, 34
dexmedetomidine, 35
etomidate and propofol, 35
induction, 35
intrathoracic surgical procedures, 36
ketamine, 34, 35
modalities, 33
monitoring, 35
nitrous oxide ($N_2O$), 35
opiates, 35
pectus deformities, 36
pediatric chest wall lesions, 33, 34
preanesthetic assessment, 33–34
regional (*see* Regional analgesia)
Aneurysmal bone cysts, 88, 89
Angiosarcoma, 94, 95
Autologous fat grafting, 66–68
Autologous tissue flaps, 97

**B**

Benign chest wall tumors
bony lesions
aneurysmal bone cysts, 88
chondromas, 87
eosinophilic granuloma/langerhans cell
histiocytosis, 87–88
fibrous dysplasia, 87
osteoblastoma, 88
osteochondroma, 87
osteoid osteomas, 88
soft tissue lesions
desmoid tumors, 90–91
elastofibromas, 91
hemangiomas, 90
intercostal hernias, 88
lipomas, 88–90
lymphangiomas, 90
neurogenic tumors, 90
Bovine hardware disease, 21
Bronchoscopy, 98

**C**

Cardiac anomalies, 72
Cervical ectopia cordis, 75
Chemotherapy
angiosarcoma, 94
chondrosarocoma, 91
Ewing sarcoma, 93
liposarcomas, 94
neoadjuvant, 91, 93, 95, 99
radiation therapy, 96
Chest wall tumors
biopsy, 85–86
diagnosis
chest radiograph, 84
CT scan, 84, 85
PET imaging, 84–86
US, 85
MRI scan, 84, 85
musculoskeletal structure, 83
preoperative evaluation, 86
reconstruction, 97–98
signs and symptoms,
83–84
surgical management, 96–97
surveillance, 98
Chondromas, 87, 89
Chondrosarcomas, 91, 94
Cryoablation, 41–42
Cryoanalgesia, 41
Currarino-Silverman syndrome, 27

© Springer International Publishing Switzerland 2017
G.W. Raff, S. Hirose (eds.), *Surgery for Chest Wall Deformities*,
DOI 10.1007/978-3-319-43926-6

**D**

Deep inferior epigastric artery perforator (DIEP) flap, 66
Desmoid tumors, 90–91
DIEP flap. *See* Deep inferior epigastric artery perforator
 (DIEP) flap

**E**

Ectopia cordis
 cervical, 75
 somatic tissue, 74
 thoracic cavity, 74
 thoraco-abdominal, 75, 76
 ventral wall defects, 74, 75
Elastofibromas, 91, 92
Eosinophilic granuloma, 87–89
Epidural analgesia, 39–40
Ewing sarcoma, 91–94
Exercise programs, 13

**F**

Fibromas, 92
Fibrosarcoma, 95
Fibrous dysplasia, 87, 89

**G**

Giant cell tumor, 89

**H**

Haller index, 11, 16
Hemangiomas, 90, 92
Hypoxic pulmonary vasoconstriction (HPV), 35

**I**

Inferior gluteal artery perforator (IGAP) flap, 66
Intercostal nerves, 5

**L**

Langerhans cell histiocytosis, 87, 88
Lipomas, 88–90, 92
Liposarcomas, 93–95
Lymphangiomas, 90, 92

**M**

Magnetic mini-mover procedure (3MP)
 axial diagram, 20
 chest wall correction, 19
 description, 15
 development and preclinical testing, 20–21
 Magnatract, 19, 20
 magnetic field, 19
 Magnimplant, 19, 20
 phase I clinical trial
  cardiac function, wound repair, bone and cartilage
   stability, 25

clinical device adaptations, 23, 24
 cost effectiveness, 23–25
 CT scans, PSI, 23
 mean compliance and PSI, 22
 safety, 22–23
 sensor data, 22
 study design, 21–22
 phase II clinical trial, 25–26
Malignant chest wall tumors
 bony lesions
  chondrosarcomas, 91
  Ewing sarcoma, 91–93
  osteosarcomas, 91
  solitary plasmacytoma, 93
 soft tissue lesions
  angiosarcoma, 94
  liposarcomas, 93–94
  MFH, 93
  radiation-associated malignant tumors, 96
  resection, metastatic cancers, 96, 97
  rhabdomyosarcoma, 94–96
  soft tissue sarcomas, 93
Malignant fibrous histiocytomas (MFH), 93, 95
Marfan syndrome, 8, 28
Mesoderm, 73
Metastatic disease, 96
Mosaicism, 49
3MP. *See* Magnetic mini-mover procedure (3MP)

**N**

Neurofibrosarcomas, 95
Neurogenic tumors, 90, 92
Non-opioid analgesia, 37
Nonsteroidal anti-inflammatory drugs (NSAIDs), 37
Noonan syndrome, 8, 28
NSAIDs. *See* Nonsteroidal anti-inflammatory drugs
 (NSAIDs)
Nursing care
 pectus carinatum, 104–105
 pectus excavatum (*see* Pectus excavatum)
 rib resection
  ambulation, 106
  cardiac and hemodynamics, 105
  chest X-rays, 105
  definition, 105
  discharge and follow-up, 106
  gastrointestinal, 106
  intensive care unit, 105
  oxygen saturations, 105
  pain control, 105
  preoperative preparation, 105
  thoracotomy, 105
Nuss procedure, 13–14, 36–38, 40
Nuss repair, 19, 26

**O**

Omphalopagus conjoined twins, 79
Opioid analgesia, 36–37
Orthotic bracing, 30

Osteoblastoma, 88
Osteochondroma, 87, 89
Osteoid osteomas, 88, 89
Osteosarcomas, 91, 94

**P**
Paravertebral block (PVB), 40
Pectus carinatum
    assessment, 28
    chondrogladiolar deformity, 27, 28
    chondromanubrial deformity, 27, 28
    defects, 27
    description, 27
    diagnosis, 28
    and excavatum, 28
    incidence, 27
    management, 29
    nonoperative repair, 30
    operative repair, 29–30
    scoliosis and spinal deformities, 28
Pectus excavatum
    anesthesia (*see* Anesthesia)
    assessment, 11
    asymmetry, 9
    cardiopulmonary impairment, 10
    cardiovascular function, 10–11
    case of, 7
    causes, 101
    chest pain, 101
    chest wall anatomy, 9
    complications, 14–15
    cryoablation, 102
    definition, 7
    echocardiogram, 101
    genetic syndromes, 8
    indications, operative repair, 11–13
    3MP (*see* Magnetic mini-mover procedure
        (3MP))
    Nuss/Ravitch procedures
        ambulation, 103
        cardiac and hemodynamics, 103
        chest X-rays, 102
        discharge and follow-up, 103–104
        gastrointestinal, 103
        Haller index, 102
        intensive care unit, 102
        pain control, 103
        pulmonary, 102–103
        timing of surgery, 102
    pathogenesis, 8
    physical features, 9
    presentation, 9
    prosthetic implants, 15
    psychological benefits, 15
    psychosocial concerns, 102
    pulmonary function, 10
    Ravitch repair, 7
    recurrence rates, 15
    repair, rib cartilage, 7
    sternal infection and necrosis, 8
        sternocostal cartilage, 9
        sternum, 8
        symptoms, 10
        systolic ejection murmur, 10
        trunk, 8
Pectus severity index (PSI), 22, 23
Pediatric anesthesia. *See* Anesthesia
Pediatric tumors, 96
Pentalogy of Cantrell, 79
Physiology, 71, 78, 80, 81
Poland's syndrome
    aesthetic deformity, 68
    anatomic dissection, 47
    bilateral muscle, 48
    breast, 57
    cadaver's thorax, 47
    chest wall
        pectoralis major muscle, 57
        pectoralis minor muscle, 57
    classification, 49
    complex form, 49
    deformities, 47
    description, 47
    diagnosis, 51–53
    incidence, 48
    pathogenesis, 48–49
    pectoralis major muscle, 49
    severity, 50
    simple form, 49
    thoracic skeleton, 54–56
    treatment, 53
Prenatal diagnosis, 51
PSI. *See* Pectus severity index (PSI)


**R**
Radiation-associated malignant tumors, 96
Radiotherapy, 88, 95
Ravitch repair, 7, 12, 13, 15, 19, 26, 30
Regional analgesia
    cryoablation, 41–42
    epidural analgesia, 39–40
    PVB, 40
    subcutaneous catheters, 40–41
Rhabdomyosarcoma, 94–96


**S**
Scapula, 5
Skeletal reconstruction, Poland's syndrome
    ADM, 63
    autologous rib grafts, 59
    breast, 59
    Fonkalsrud procedure, 58
    methacrylate prosthesis, 62
    Nuss procedure, 58
    Ravitch procedure, 58
    rib hypoplasia, 59
    silicone gel prostheses, 62
    synthetic patches/meshes, 62
    thoracic skeletal deformity, 59

Soft tissue reconstruction, Poland's syndrome
    autologous fat grafting, 66–68
    flap alone, 65–66
    implant with flap, 65
    implant-alone approach, 64–65
Soft tissue sarcomas, 93, 95
Solitary plasmacytoma, 93, 94
Sternal anatomy
    abdominal wall and liver, 79
    development, 71, 72
    diagnosis, 73
    ectopia cordis (*see* Ectopia cordis)
    sternal clefts, 73–74
    sternal defects, 72
Sternal clefts
    anterior chest wall anomalies, 78–79
    bifid sternum, 77
    congenital anomalies, 73
    CT scan, 79
    endothoracic fascia, 77
    neonatal period, 76
    primary repair, 76, 77
    surgical repair, 73, 74
    syndromes, 73
    ultrasound, 71
Sternal defects, 72
Sternal development, 71, 72
Sternal fractures, 80
Sternal infections, 80–81
Sternal suction device, 13
Sternum
    carinatum defect, 28
    costal cartilages and osteotomy, 7
    depression, 9, 10
    intrauterine pressure, 8
    magnet field, 25
    manubrium, 1, 8
    mesenchymal bands, 8
    ossification, 8
    osteotomy, 29
    ribs and cartilage, 8
    sternal body, 1, 8
    structure, intercostal space, 1
    titanium-encased anterior magnet, 25
    xiphoid process, 1
    xyphoid process, 23
Subclavian artery supply disruption sequence
        (SASDS), 49
Subcutaneous catheters, 40–41
Superficial inferior epigastric artery (SIEA) flap, 66
Superior gluteal artery perforator (SGAP) flap, 66


**T**
Thoracic anesthesia. *See* Anesthesia
Thoraco-abdominal ectopia cordis, 75, 76
Thoracodorsal artery perforator (TDAP) flap, 66
Thoracopagus twins, 79–80
Thorax
    intercostal muscles and spaces, 4–5
    neurovascular anatomy, 4
    Poland's syndrome, 5
    respiration, muscles, 5
    ribs, 2–4
    sternum, 1–2
TRAM flap. *See* Transverse rectus abdominus
        myocutaneous (TRAM) flap
Transverse myocutaneous gracilis (TMG) flap, 66
Transverse rectus abdominus myocutaneous (TRAM)
        flap, 66


**X**
Xiphoid process, 1